T0297692

Endocrine Disruptors and
The Developing Brain

Colloquium Series on The Developing Brain

Editor
Margaret M. McCarthy, Ph.D.
Professor and Chair
Department of Pharmacology
University of Maryland School of Medicine

The goal of this series is to provide a comprehensive state-of-the-art overview of how the brain develops and those processes that affect it. Topics range from the fundamentals of axonal guidance and synaptogenesis prenatally to the influence of hormones, sex, stress, maternal care, and injury during the early postnatal period to an additional critical period at puberty. Easily accessible expert reviews combine analyses of detailed cellular mechanisms with interpretations of significance and broader impact of the topic area on the field of neuroscience and the understanding of brain and behavior.

My research program focuses on the influence of steroid hormones on the developing brain. During perinatal life, there is a sensitive period for hormone exposure during which permanent cytoarchitectural changes are established. Males and females are exposed to different hormonal milieus and this results in sex differences in the brain. These differences include alterations in the volumes of particular brain nuclei and patterns of synaptic connectivity. The mechanisms by which sexually dimorphic structures are formed in the brain remains poorly understood.

I received my PhD in Behavioral and Neural Sciences from the Institute of Animal Behavior at Rutgers University in Newark, NJ in 1989. I then spent three years as a post-doctoral fellow at the Rockefeller University in New York, NY and one year as a National Research Council Fellow at the National Institutes of Health, before joining the faculty at the University of Maryland. I am a member of the University of Maryland Graduate School and the Center for Studies in Reproduction. I am also a member of the Society for Behavioral Neuroendocrinology, the Society for Neuroscience, the American Physiological Association, and the Endocrine Society.

Copyright © 2012 by Morgan & Claypool Life Sciences

All rights reserved. No part of this publication may be reproduced, stored in a retrieval system, or transmitted in any form or by any means—electronic, mechanical, photocopy, recording, or any other except for brief quotations in printed reviews, without the prior permission of the publisher.

Endocrine Disruptors and The Developing Brain
Andrea C. Gore and Sarah M. Dickerson
www.morganclaypool.com

ISBN: 9781615040872 paperback

ISBN: 9781615040889 ebook

DOI: 10.4199/C00054ED1V01Y201204DBR007

A Publication in the

COLLOQUIUM SERIES ON THE DEVELOPING BRAIN

Lecture #7

Series Editor: Margaret M. McCarthy, University of Maryland School of Medicine

Series ISSN

ISSN   2159-5194   print
ISSN   2159-5208   electronic

Endocrine Disruptors and The Developing Brain

Andrea C. Gore and Sarah M. Dickerson
The University of Texas at Austin
Division of Pharmacology and Toxicology

COLLOQUIUM SERIES ON THE DEVELOPING BRAIN # 7

MORGAN&CLAYPOOL LIFE SCIENCES

ABSTRACT

The field of endocrine disruption has been the focus of increasing attention from scientists and the general public in the past 30 years, amidst concerns that exposure to environmental chemicals with the potential to alter endocrine system function, known as endocrine disrupting chemicals (EDCs), may be contributing to an overall decline in wildlife populations and the reproductive health of humans. These concerns are based on observations of adverse effects of EDCs on marine and land animals, an increased incidence of reproductive and endocrine disease in humans, epidemiological evidence for links between body burden and disease, and endocrine disruption in laboratory animals following exposure to EDCs. Owing to its role in regulation of endocrine function as well as its responsiveness to hormones, the developing brain is an especially vulnerable target for many classes of EDCs. This book will address the evidence for EDC action on the developing brain, organized into 7 chapters. Topics covered include background about EDCs, evidence for exposures, concerns about EDC effects in the developing organism, and particularly on the developing nervous system, how EDCs perturb the brain's neuroendocrine systems, transgenerational epigenetic effects of EDCs, EDC effects on non-reproductive behaviors, and future perspectives. This is the first book completely dedicated to understanding links between EDCs and the developing brain, an area of emerging importance for human health.

KEYWORDS

endocrine disrupting chemical (EDC), brain sexual differentiation, fetal basis of adult disease, developmental toxicology, estrogen, GnRH, hormone, hypothalamus, nervous system, testosterone

Contents

1. **What Are Environmental Endocrine-Disrupting Chemicals (EDCs)?** 1
   1.1 Introduction to EDCs 1
   1.2 Endocrine Systems Communicate with the Environment 3
   1.3 Hormonal Properties and Mechanisms of EDCs................................... 4
       1.3.1 Nuclear Hormone Receptors... 4
       1.3.2 Membrane Hormone Receptors 8
       1.3.3 Steroidogenic Enzymes 9
   1.4 Representative EDCs and their Actions... 10
       1.4.1 Industrial Organohalogens (PCBs, PBDEs)............................. 11
       1.4.2 Pesticides (DDT, methoxychlor)... 12
       1.4.3 Phytoestrogens 13
   1.5 Summary and Conclusions... 15

2. **EDC Exposures** 17
   2.1 EDCs and Wildlife 17
       2.1.1 Reproductive Toxicity of EDCs in Wildlife 20
   2.2 EDCs and Humans 21
       2.2.1 Diethylstilbestrol (DES).. 23
       2.2.2 PCBs 23
       2.2.3 Dioxins 24
       2.2.4 Low-Dose Human Exposures: What Is the Evidence?............. 24
   2.3 Summary and Conclusions... 25

3. **EDCs and Development**...27
   3.1 Vulnerability of the Developing Fetus 27
   3.2 Fetal (Developmental) Basis of Adult Disease 27
   3.3 Critical Developmental Periods.. 28

3.4   Key Toxicological Principles Relevant to Developmental Exposures.................. 29
    3.4.1   LOAEL/NOAEL 29
    3.4.2   Dose–Response Principles and Why they Do Not Apply to EDCs...... 30
    3.4.3   Low-Dose Effects of EDCs—Lack of a Threshold 31
3.5   Summary and Conclusions.. 33

4.   **EDCs and the Developing Brain**... **35**
4.1   Hormones and Brain Sexual Differentiation 35
    4.1.1   Hormones and Neuronal Survival and Death 36
4.2   EDCs and the Perturbation of Brain Sexual Differentiation................. 38
    4.2.1   Hypothalamic Morphology.. 38
    4.2.2   Hypothalamic Developmental Apoptosis.................................... 39
    4.2.3   Neuronal Phenotype... 39
4.3   EDCs and Reproductive Behaviors... 41
4.4   EDCs and Non-Reproductive Behaviors 43
    4.4.1   Hormones and Synaptic Plasticity... 44
    4.4.2   EDCs and Neural Plasticity 44
    4.4.3   EDC Effects on the Brain's Dopamine Neurons 45
4.5   Summary and Conclusions.. 46

5.   **EDCs and Neuroendocrine Systems**.. **49**
5.1   Neuroendocrine Systems of the Hypothalamus................................... 49
5.2   Reproductive Neuroendocrine Systems and Perturbations by EDCs................ 53
    5.2.1   Background on GnRH Neurons.. 53
    5.2.2   Sexual Differentiation of the HPG Axis 56
    5.2.3   Steroid Hormone Feedback and Regulation of HPG Function 57
    5.2.4   Disruption of GnRH Neurons by EDCs 59
        5.2.4.1   *In vitro* Evidence 59
        5.2.4.2   *In vivo* Evidence 60
        5.2.4.3   Developmental EDC Exposures and GnRH Neurons..........61
    5.2.5   EDCs, Puberty, and the Brain.. 62
        5.2.5.1   Disruption of Puberty by Environmental EDCs....................63
        5.2.5.2   Kisspeptin Neurons Are Potential Targets for
                    Developmental EDCs 64
5.3   Summary and Conclusions.. 64

6.   Epigenetic Effects of EDCs 67

　6.1   Molecular Epigenetic Mechanisms: An Introduction 67

　6.2   Hormones and Epigenetic Change 69

　　　6.2.1   DNA Methylation.. 69

　　　6.2.2   Histone Modifications... 70

　　　6.2.3   MicroRNAs.. 70

　6.3   Transgenerational Epigenetic Effects of EDCs.................................. 71

　　　6.3.1   Vinclozolin 71

　　　6.3.2   Bisphenol A... 72

　　　6.3.3   Diethylstilbesterol (DES) 73

　　　6.3.4   Polychlorinated Biphenyls (PCBs) 74

　　　6.3.5   Methoxychlor 74

　6.4   The Importance of Context in Environmental Epigenetics 75

　6.5   Summary and Conclusions.. 75

7.   EDCs, the Brain, and the Future 77

　7.1   Can EDC Effects Be Mitigated?... 77

　7.2   What Can We Do to Avoid EDC Exposures?.................................... 79

　7.3   General Conclusions 82

Acknowledgments.. 85

References 87

Author Biographies... 99

CHAPTER 1

What Are Environmental Endocrine-Disrupting Chemicals (EDCs)?

1.1 INTRODUCTION TO EDCs

We live in an increasingly man-made world. There are currently more than 85,000 chemicals used for industrial purposes, and it is virtually impossible to avoid contact with hundreds of chemicals every day. Some of these chemicals are toxic, causing adverse health effects. Others do not cause overt toxic effects, but may induce subtle changes that over time lead to increased propensity for physiological dysfunctions. We are exposed to chemicals through the air we breathe, our food and water, clothing, soil, dust, and the consumer products we use. In fact, the Centers for Disease Control and Prevention (CDC) can detect very small levels of more than 300 such chemicals in human blood and urine. Some of these compounds are endocrine-disrupting chemicals (EDCs; Table 1). We define EDCs as any exogenous compound that causes changes to hormonal systems and their actions.

The chemical revolution began in the 1940s, making this the third generation exposed to increasing numbers and levels of industrial chemicals (Crews and Gore, 2011). Considering how many of these compounds come into contact with the food that we eat, the water we drink, are applied to our skin, or are in our clothing and furniture, it is surprising that governmental regulatory bodies have not carefully monitored their potential biological effects. Nevertheless, the topic of environmental exposures and public health risk has become the focus of increasing attention from scientists, the media, and the general public. The evidence for adverse effects of environmental EDCs is growing. In animals, wildlife populations with known EDC exposures demonstrate consequences on reproduction and behavior (Markman et al., 2008). Laboratory animal models, particularly rodents and also primates, demonstrate effects of EDCs on virtually every endocrine system studied. There is also increasing evidence for effects of EDCs on neurobiological development and on a variety of behaviors, both reproductive and non-reproductive (Schantz and Widholm, 2001; Steinberg et al., 2007).

In humans, there is greater controversy, due to the enormous variability in populations, exposures, and endpoints examined (Luoma, 2005). There are a few good (albeit unfortunate) examples of human exposures. Cooking oil contamination by industrial chemicals now known to be endocrine disruptors (polychlorinated biphenyls), release of dioxin into the environment due to a factory explosion in Seveso, Italy, and other high-dose exposures showed not only acute toxic effects but

TABLE 1: Common sources of EDCs		
SOURCE	CLASS(ES) OF EDC(S)	EXAMPLES
Plants	Phytoestrogens	Alfalfa, red clover, soy, fruits, nuts, whole grains, vegetables, flaxseed, fungus, mold
Fresh Produce	Pesticide residues	Celery, peaches, cherries, apples, domestic blueberries, nectarines, sweet bell peppers, strawberries, potatoes, grapes, spinach, kale and collard greens, lettuce
Fish	PCBs, DDT, mercury	Salmon, tuna, shark, king mackerel, marlin, orange roughy
Air	Various semi-volatile and volatile EDCs	Smog, particulate matter, aerosols, dust
Water	Water-soluble EDCs	Surface water, treated waste water, drinking water-contaminated with such EDCs as pesticides, industrial chemicals, ethinyl estradiol (oral contraceptive), phenols
Soil and sediments	PCBs, dioxins, PBDEs	Topsoil, sewage sludge, leachate from landfills
Plastics	Bisphenol A (BPA), Phthalates	Disposable plastic water bottles and food containers, medical tubing
Pesticides, Herbicides	Organohalogenated compounds	DDT, lindane, methoxychlor, vinclozolin
Consumer Products	Various EDCs	Cosmetics, cleaning products, personal care products, sunscreens, garden chemicals

also longer-lasting effects consistent with the endocrine-disrupting properties of these chemicals, defined in more detail below.

1.2 ENDOCRINE SYSTEMS COMMUNICATE WITH THE ENVIRONMENT

In order to understand the actions of EDCs on the brain, it is first necessary to provide some brief background on the anatomy and physiology of endocrine systems. The endocrine system is one of three major systems (the others being the nervous and immune) that enable the body to communicate with, and respond to, the environment. Endocrine organs are defined by the release of

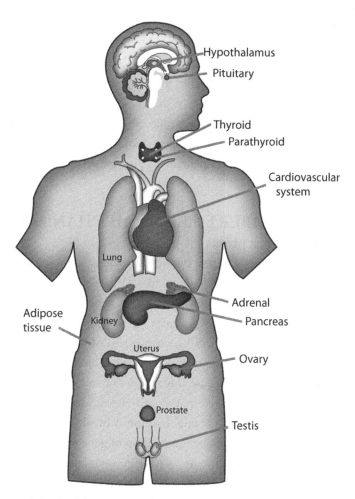

FIGURE 1: Many of the body's major endocrine systems are shown. Modified from Diamanti-Kandarakis et al. (2009).

chemical signals (hormones) into the blood system, followed by transport to a target organ where the hormone can act upon specific receptors. A subset of endocrine systems in the body is shown in Figure 1. There are many more glands not shown that have endocrine or mixed endocrine functions, including the pineal, placenta, liver, stomach, intestines, bone, skin, and others.

The hormones produced by endocrine glands can be peptides, proteins, steroids, or catecholamines. Hormones signal through receptors localized in target tissues, and there are hormone receptors in the G-protein coupled, cytokine, and nuclear receptor families, each with unique distributions in the body. As an example of endocrine signaling, the pancreas produces several classes of protein hormones, including insulin and glucagon, whose receptors are widely distributed in order to maintain glucose levels. Notably, the bulk of the pancreas serves non-endocrine functions involved in digestion, illustrating the fact that some glands have mixed endocrine and non-endocrine functions.

The gonads and adrenals produce steroid hormones, as well as protein and catecholamine (adrenal only) hormones, through release into the blood system. In the case of the adrenal, different tissue zones of the adrenal gland produce catecholamines (epinephrine and norepinephrine from the adrenal medulla); the adrenal cortex produces glucocorticoids (stress hormones), mineralocorticoids (electrolyte balance, blood pressure), and sex steroids, especially dehydroepiandrosterone (DHEA). This illustrates the point that one gland many produce many hormones, often many types of hormones.

1.3 HORMONAL PROPERTIES AND MECHANISMS OF EDCs

1.3.1 Nuclear Hormone Receptors

The steroid hormone family includes gonadal steroids (estrogens, androgens, and progestins) and adrenal steroids (glucocorticoids and mineralocorticoids). When one of these hormones is synthesized, it is released and transported through the circulatory system. At the appropriate target organ, binding of the steroid hormone to its specific receptor results in intracellular interactions between the steroid–receptor complex with specific DNA sequences, called hormone response elements. Together with other proteins in the cell that are recruited by ligand binding, this complex activates the transcription of the DNA target gene. Because this manner of steroid signaling occurs within the cell nucleus, these steroid hormones are referred to as "nuclear" steroid hormone receptors, and the mode of signaling is referred to as "genomic" because it involves interactions of the steroid–receptor complex with DNA and the subsequent activation of gene expression. For example, binding of estrogens to the estrogen receptor in some tissues can result in activation of target DNA that transcribes the progesterone receptor, leading to up-regulation of progesterone receptor protein in these cells.

TABLE 2: Summary of common EDC mechanisms of action

RECEPTOR-MEDIATED MECHANISMS FOR EDC ACTION

A. Nuclear Hormone Receptors

Receptor	Endogenous ligand	Function	Examples of EDCs
Androgen (AR)	Testosterone	Male reproductive function, behavior	Phthalates Pesticides
Estrogen (ER) α & β	Estradiol	Female reproductive cycle, function, behavior	Alkylphenols BPA DES Dioxins EE Furans Halogenated hydrocarbons
Peroxisome proliferator–activated receptor (PPARγ)	Free fatty acids Eicosanoids	Lipid homeostasis, Adipogenesis, Metabolism	Organotin compounds
Progesterone (PR)	Progesterone	Female reproductive cycle, function, behavior	BPA Pesticides
Retinoid (RXR)	Retinoic acid	Lipid homeostasis, adipogenesis	Arsenic Organotin compounds

TABLE 2: (*continued*)

RECEPTOR-MEDIATED MECHANISMS FOR EDC ACTION

A. Nuclear Hormone Receptors

Receptor	Endogenous ligand	Function	Examples of EDCs
Thyroid (TR) α & β	Thyroid hormone	Metabolism	BPA Dioxins PBDEs PCBs Perchlorates Pesticides Phthalates

B. Non-nuclear hormone receptors

Receptor	Endogenous ligand	Function	Examples of EDCs
Membrane estrogen (mER, GPR30)	Estradiol	Cell differentiation, survival, proliferation	BPA cadmium
Membrane progesterone (mPR)	Progesterone	Cell differentiation and proliferation	DES

Arylhydrocarbon (AhR)	Unknown	Development, xenobiotic metabolism	Dioxins Dioxin-like PCBs TCDD
Neurotransmitter receptors (serotonin, dopamine, norepinephrine, etc.)	Neurotransmitters (5-HT, DA, NE, etc.)	Regulatory input onto neuroendocrine systems	PCBs

NON-RECEPTOR-MEDIATED MECHANISMS FOR EDC ACTION

Mechanism	Example EDCs
Decreased androgen synthesis	Phthalates (*DEHP, DBP, BBP*)
Altered brain aromatase levels	PCBs, atrazine
Steroid synthesis inhibition	Ketoconazole
Interference with steroid metabolism via estrogen sulfotransferase inhibition	PCBs

From an historical standpoint, some of the earliest reports of endocrine disruption came from farmers who noted that sheep feeding on red clover fields became infertile. Scientists later discovered that clover contains phytoestrogens, a class of compounds produced by many plants that could mimic the actions of endogenous estrogen by virtue of their chemical structure. This property is known as estrogenicity, although we now know that EDCs can also be anti-estrogenic, androgenic (mimicking the actions of endogenous androgens such as testosterone), or anti-androgenic in nature. To date, estrogenic endocrine disruptors are the most common, possibly due to properties of the estrogen receptor that enable it to interact with ligands that are seemingly "un-estrogenic" in structure but nevertheless can exert estrogenic functions. Since the time of these early observations, hundreds of synthetic chemicals have been identified as endocrine disruptors.

The EDCs we encounter daily in our environment act to imitate, block, or otherwise interfere with endogenous endocrine activity. Some of the known mechanisms (Table 2) through which hormonal function may be compromised include direct or indirect interaction of EDCs with steroid hormone receptors. Some EDCs have structural similarity to the body's endogenous hormones and can bind to hormone receptors. Along with their effects on estrogen receptors, other steroid hormone receptors, such as androgen and progesterone receptors, are potential targets. Thyroid hormone receptors, while not members of the steroid hormone receptor superfamily, are also nuclear receptors that can bind to certain EDCs, which act as agonists or antagonists. In general, EDCs bind to steroid hormone receptors with lower affinity than do our endogenous hormones; nevertheless, they still have the capacity to activate the same transcriptional processes acted upon by our natural hormones.

1.3.2 Membrane Hormone Receptors

There are several classes of membrane steroid receptors that are potential targets of EDCs. Some membrane steroid receptors are identical to the nuclear receptors, but instead of existing within the cell (in the nucleus and/or cytoplasm), they are associated with cell membranes. Other membrane steroid hormone receptors are structurally distinct from the nuclear receptors. These membrane proteins are generally referred to as membrane estrogen receptors (mER), membrane progesterone receptors (mPR), and membrane androgen receptors (mAR), several of which have been cloned. For this type of membrane-mediated signaling, steroid hormones do not need to diffuse through the membrane; rather, their interaction with receptors occurs at the level of the membrane itself. Instead of the receptor–ligand complex binding directly to DNA, the membrane steroid hormone receptors signal through other intracellular pathways such as those involving calcium flux, protein phosphorylation, cyclic AMP, MAP kinases, and other signaling molecules. These types of signal transduction pathways are very rapid and are consistent with the earlier observations for effects of steroid hormones occurring within seconds.

In the nervous system, recent research has focused on a membrane estrogen receptor called GPER (also called GPR30). Binding of estrogens to GPER and other membrane hormone receptors in the brain are associated with neural signaling involving depolarization and neurotransmitter release. There is also a membrane PR, called Pgrmc1, which is highly abundant in nervous tissue and speculated to be involved in the rapid effects of progestins in the brain.

1.3.3 Steroidogenic Enzymes

Steroid hormone biosynthesis begins with the cholesterol molecule precursor. Through a series of enzymatic conversions, steroidogenesis (the biosynthesis of steroids) leads to the production of active steroids as well as processing intermediates (Figure 2). The common cholesterol precursor is, therefore, the starting point for progesterone, testosterone, estradiol, aldosterone, and cortisol. Steroidogenesis is highly conserved across mammals and even across vertebrates. Two steroidogenic

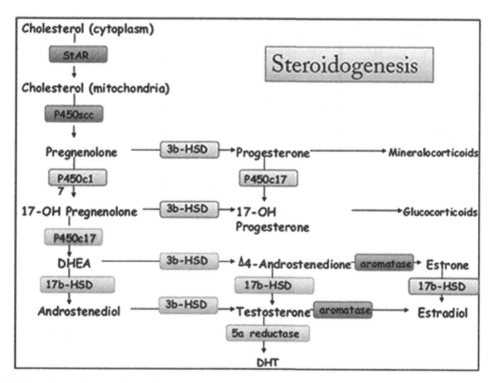

FIGURE 2: Steroidogenesis begins with conversion of cholesterol by a series of enzymatic reactions into the mineralocorticoids, glucocorticoids and sex steroids. The focus of this figure is on sex steroid biosynthesis, showing key hormones and intermediates, and enzymes involved in these processes. From McCarthy (2011).

enzymes, p450 aromatase (aromatase), which converts androgens to estrogens, and 5α-reductase, which reduces testosterone to a more potent androgen, dihydrotestosterone (**DHT**), are crucial for biosynthesis and metabolism of androgens and estrogens and are particularly important in the context of EDCs. There is strong evidence that depending upon the specific EDC, the target tissue, and the developmental stage of exposure, EDCs can stimulate or inhibit gene expression or activity of steroidogenic enzymes, with concomitant effects on levels of estrogens and androgens. EDCs, including atrazine, BPA, phthalates, and triclosan, are known to have steroidogenic effects.

1.4   REPRESENTATIVE EDCs AND THEIR ACTIONS

The following sections of this chapter will highlight three representative classes of EDCs, chosen because they are known to target the brain and, more specifically, neuroendocrine systems: phytoestrogens, industrial organohalogens, and pesticides, representative structures of which are shown in Figure 3.

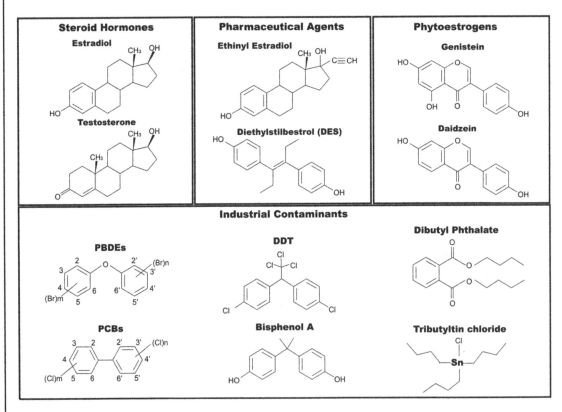

FIGURE 3: Structures of representative EDCs.

1.4.1 Industrial Organohalogens (PCBs, PBDEs)

Industrial organohalogens are an array of synthetic halogen-containing organic compounds that are used for or produced as a byproduct of commercial applications. Included in this diverse class of contaminants are plastic polymers, dioxins, polychlorinated biphenyls (PCBs), polybrominated diphenyl ether flame-retardants (PBDEs), chlorinated paraffins, and furans. Members of this class of toxicants are generally stable and resistant to degradation. As a result, once they get into an organism, they typically bioaccumulate in the tissues of exposed organisms, and they biomagnify across the foodchain. In fact, they are routinely detected in samples from humans and wildlife. Exposure to this class of compounds typically occurs via consumption of contaminated foods such as farm-raised salmon. The levels of PCBs and other EDCs in farm-raised salmon (Hites et al., 2004) have prompted public health officials to advise pregnant women to limit their consumption of this otherwise healthy food option to once monthly.

Although there are many compounds in this category of EDCs, much of the data regarding the effects of industrial organohalogens on the developing brain, as will be discussed later, comes from studies with PCBs (Figure 3), a family of 209 compounds that share in common a biphenyl core and differ in the number and arrangement of chlorine atoms. This structural feature facilitates their interaction with various hormone and neurotransmitter receptors, where they may act as agonists, antagonists, or with mixed activity. For instance, the phenolic moiety of endogenous estradiol binds to estrogen receptors, an interaction that is mimicked by PCBs and other phenolic EDCs.

PCBs were used widely between the 1930s and 1970s for such industrial applications as capacitors, transformer oil, sealants, paints, etc., but their manufacture was banned in 1977 due to their toxicity. More than three decades later, they are still prevalent environmental contaminants found in sediments and marine biota. The chemical properties that made PCBs ideal for industry, namely, their structural stability and resistance to degradation, made them persistent in the environment, bioaccumulate in fatty tissues of exposed organisms, and biomagnify in the food chain. Migration of contaminated organisms due to climate fluctuation, as well as air and water currents carry PCBs to even remote areas such as the Arctic and Antarctic, where they are found as complex mixtures of the most persistent congeners and their hydroxylated metabolites.

PCBs are classified into one of the following three categories: coplanar, dioxin-like coplanar, or non-coplanar, based upon their three-dimensional structure (Dickerson et al., 2012). PCBs interact with hormone and neurotransmitter receptors as agonists, antagonists, or with mixed activity, depending largely upon their structural properties. For example, PCBs may be estrogenic, anti-estrogenic, or anti-androgenic. PCBs target a whole host of receptors including hormone receptors (estrogen, androgen, thyroid), neurotransmitter receptors (acetylcholine, dopamine, GABA, and serotonin), orphan receptors (aryl hydrocarbon), as well as hormone-binding proteins, intracellular signaling molecules and receptors (ryanodine receptor), and enzymes that metabolize hormones, such as estrogen sulfotransferase (Dickerson et al., 2012). Furthermore, additivity, synergy, or antagonistic effects between different PCBs may occur in the complex mixtures typically found in environmental, animal, and human samples.

1.4.2 Pesticides (DDT, methoxychlor)

Of all the EDC classes discussed in this section, pesticides have the longest history and largest scale of global use due to their wide range of agricultural, commercial, and residential pest control applications. Often classified according to the organism targeted (Table 3), pesticides include insecticides, herbicides, and fungicides, which target unwanted insects, plants, and fungi, respectively. Although their utility in the eradication of disease vectors and targeted pests is unquestionable, pesticides also have unintended actions on the developing brain and endocrine systems of non-targeted species, including humans, even at very low levels.

Alternatively, pesticides can be classified as chemical pesticides (synthetic, i.e., carbamate, organochlorine, organophosphorus, pyrethroid) or biopesticides (derived from natural sources). Although there are several classes of chemical pesticides, the organochlorine and organophosphate families have been the most studied from an endocrine disruption perspective. Like halogenated

TABLE 3: Types of pesticides classified according to targeted species	
CLASS OF PESTICIDE	**TARGETED SPECIES**
Algicides	Algae
Avicides	Birds
Bactericides	Bacteria
Fungicides	Fungi (mildew, molds, rusts)
Insecticides	Insects
Molluscicides	Molluscs
Nematicides	Nematodes
Rodenticides	Rodents

organic compounds, organochlorine pesticides are lipophilic, partitioning into the body's fat stores, where they remain for years. Humans are primarily exposed to organochlorine pesticides through direct skin contact or inhalation during pest control and/or via consumption of residues on fruits and vegetables. Organochlorine insecticides include such agents as dichlorodiphenyltrichloroethane (DDT; Figure 3), methoxychlor, dicofol, heptachlor, chlordane, endosulfan, aldrin, dieldrin, endrin, and mirex.

In the 1970s, emerging scientific evidence linking organochlorine pesticide exposure to adverse effects in humans and wildlife populations prompted a ban on many pesticides in this class, including DDT. DDT and other organochlorine pesticides such as dieldrin, kepone, and methoxychlor are weakly estrogenic, although some have also been found to possess anti-estrogenic and/or anti-androgenic activities. Moreover, organochlorine pesticides may exert indirect effects on neuroendocrine function through their actions on neurotransmitter synthesis/degradation and/or receptors, some of which have inputs to the hypothalamus (e.g., cholinergic, GABAergic, dopamine). Currently, there is debate between the risks and benefits of powerful pesticides such as DDT. In countries where malaria is abundant, DDT is an extremely effective pesticide. The trade-offs between malaria prevention, with high mortality, compared to endocrine-disrupting effects of DDT, are difficult to reconcile. Of course, ideally, malaria can be fought with non-chemical approaches such as the use of mosquito netting in homes.

Organophosphorus pesticides are a class of less persistent, albeit more acutely toxic compounds that replaced organochlorine pesticides. While these chemicals are not lipophilic and degrade more readily than organochlorine pesticides, humans are routinely exposed to organophosporus pesticides through contact with contaminated surfaces and consumption of contaminated produce, air, and water because they are applied ubiquitously. Organophosphorus pesticides include such agents as chlorpyrifos (now banned in the U.S.), parathion, malathion, diazinon, and dichlorvos. Although their effects on the thyroid axis have been reported, the impact of organophosphorus pesticides on reproductive neuroendocrine endpoints has not been rigorously studied and merits further investigation.

1.4.3   Phytoestrogens

Although endocrine disruption is thought to be a relatively recent discipline, the earliest studies in the field were published more than a half century ago on breeding difficulty in sheep and other livestock feeding on red clover pastures as mentioned above. Similar as effects of other plant extracts were later observed in other species, including wildlife, such as quail and deer mice, as well as laboratory animals, such as rats and mice. In addition to being a source of nutrition, researchers found that certain non-steroidal plant compounds, collectively termed phytoestrogens, were similar to the body's own estrogens in structure and action and thus could behave as weak estrogen mimics or as anti-estrogens. For example, *in vitro* binding studies showed that phytoestrogens bind to and activate the estrogen receptor (**ER**), albeit with binding affinities several orders of magnitude lower than endogenous estrogens (Kuiper et al., 1998). However, despite their low relative ER binding affinity, phytoestrogens can have a dramatic impact upon reproductive physiology, especially when exposure occurs during development.

The typical route of exposure is through the diet, as phytoestrogens are contained in a number of edible plants, including vegetables, herbs, soy, alfalfa, fruits, nuts, flax seed, nutritional supplements, wine, as well as in soy-based infant formula and baby food (Table 4). The public perception of phytoestrogens tends to be positive, and, given their natural origins, the general assumption is

TABLE 4: Phytoestrogens and their sources

CLASS	EXAMPLE COMPOUNDS	SOURCES
Isoflavonoids		
Coumestans	Coumestrol	Alfalfa, clover
Isoflavones	Daidzein, Genistein, Glycitein	Soybeans, tofu, soy nuts, chickpeas, alfalfa sprouts
	Biochanin A	Chickpeas, peanuts, alfalfa sprouts
	Formononetin Glycosides	Red clover
Flavones	Luteolin	Celery, parsley, carrots, thyme, rosemary
Flavanoids		
Flavanols	Catechins	Green tea, red wine, chocolate, apples
	Quercetin	Tea, red onion, capers, citrus
Lignans		
Lignans	Lariciresinol	Flax seed, sesame seed
	Pinoresinol	Sesame seed, rye, oat bran
	Secoisolariciresinol	Flax seed
Stilbenes		
	Resveratrol	Grapes, red wine, peanuts

that they must be beneficial to health. To be sure, a diet rich in fruits and vegetables is a healthy choice. However, it should be noted that because phytoestrogens share similar cellular and molecular targets with synthetic EDCs, they may also share deleterious effects on reproductive physiology in common with industrial EDCs (Patisaul and Jefferson, 2010). Phytoestrogen-containing dietary supplements should be taken cautiously to avoid excess consumption, as amounts of compounds are often variable and sometimes much higher than the amount indicated by the label in non-FDA-regulated supplements.

As they are diverse in chemical structure, phytoestrogens are grouped into several classes, including the flavones (e.g., luteolin), isoflavones (e.g., genistein, daidzein), flavanols (e.g., catechin), lignans (e.g., pinoresinol), and coumestans (e.g., coumestrol). Owing to structural differences, phytoestrogens have disparate actions at the ER. For example, isoflavones such as genistein and daidzein bind to both estrogen receptors ER alpha (ERα) and ER beta (ERβ) equally, although their binding affinity is several orders of magnitude lower than that of endogenous estradiol. Other phytoestrogens, such as resveratrol, bind to ERβ with 10-fold greater affinity compared to ERα, while the reverse is true for other phytoestrogens. Phytoestrogen endocrine action is not limited to their interactions with the ER. They have also been shown to increase circulating sex hormone-binding globulins, modulate enzymatic activity of steroidogenic enzymes, act as anti-oxidants, and alter signal transduction. Moreover, phytoestrogens have an effect on neuroendocrine reproductive physiology across the life cycle, and their effects are more pronounced when exposure occurs during development.

1.5   SUMMARY AND CONCLUSIONS

This first chapter has provided an overview of the anatomy and physiology of the endocrine system and a brief introduction to EDCs, including their most common sources and the mechanisms through which they exert actions in the body. Future chapters will build upon the framework of general background provided here and will focus on the actions of EDCs on the developing brain. During the fetal and early postnatal period, the brain is transformed from a set of instructions encoded in genes, to a highly complex organ comprised of specialized cells that coordinate together to direct growth and functioning of bodily systems and respond to inputs from the environment. Cells are instructed to differentiate (or even die), migrate to their appropriate location, and form linkages with other brain cells and body regions via hormonal signals. As you will learn in the following chapters, because these formative processes lay the groundwork for adult function and behavior, any disruption could potentially manifest as a diminution in an organism's capacity to survive and reproduce.

·   ·   ·   ·

CHAPTER 2

EDC Exposures

2.1   EDCs AND WILDLIFE

EDC exposures are ubiquitous. The world has been contaminated both locally and globally (Crews and Gore, 2011). Even parts of the world that never experienced any industry or local contamination have been affected by air and water currents, migratory species, and through biomagnification up the food chain. Thus, all species (including humans) are exposed worldwide to a variety of EDCs (Table 5). The recognition of effects of EDCs in wildlife first received widespread attention with the publication of Rachel Carson's *Silent Spring* in 1962. The near extinction of the American bald eagle due to the buildup of DDT (a pesticide), prompted a new recognition of the risks of exposure to chemicals that were released into the environment without consideration for toxic effects in unintended species.

Biomagnification is the process through which the concentration of a persistent contaminant increases up the food chain (Figure 4). The example of the American bald eagle, above, shows how a top predator could accumulate DDT in its body not through direct exposure but through consumption of species lower in the food chain—which in turn consumed species even lower down that were directly exposed to DDT. Marine mammals are also at the top of the food chain and include dolphins, porpoises, sea lions, seals, and whales. Through consumption of contaminated prey, organochlorine contaminants and other lipophilic chemicals accumulate in their fat stores and can be transferred to nursing young through mother's milk. Such an example of EDC exposure in mammals comes from Baltic seals exposed to organochlorines (PCBs, DDT, DDE). Populations of these species have declined as a result of disrupted immune and reproductive function. Polar bears, which consume sea mammals, have the highest concentrations of these contaminants.

Adverse effects caused by these exposures range from subtle changes in reproductive physiology and behavior to permanently altered sexual differentiation (Table 6), overt toxicity, behavioral change, and many other endocrine perturbations. Some of the observed adverse effects are exerted through known endocrine mechanisms, although, in many cases, a causal link between exposure and endocrine disruption is unclear.

TABLE 5: Examples of environmental EDC exposures in wildlife

COMPOUND (SUSPECTED OR KNOWN)	SPECIES/LOCATION	EFFECT	STRENGTH OF EVIDENCE FOR HYPOTHESIS	UNDERSTANDING OF EVIDENCE FOR EDC MECHANISM
DDT, organochlorine pesticides	American Alligator/Lake Apopka, Florida	Reproductive abnormalities	Moderate	Moderate
DDT	Birds of prey (eagles, falcons, hawks, osprey, pelicans)/USA	Eggshell thinning	Strong	Moderate
Organochlorine pesticides	Seals/Baltic Sea region	Marked population reduction presumably due to impaired reproductive and immune function	Strong	Moderate
Tributyltin	Marine gastropods	Imposex, Population reduction	Strong	Strong
Estrogenic contaminants in sewage treatment plant effluent	Fish/UK	Vitellogenin induction	Strong	Strong
Dioxins and coplanar PCBs	Trout/Lake Ontario	Developmental and reproductive abnormalities	Strong	Weak

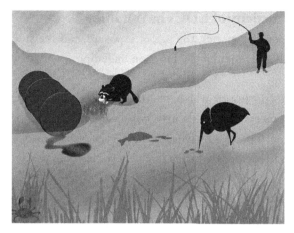

FIGURE 4: Biomagnification of persistent EDCs up the foodchain.

TABLE 6: Examples of adverse effects caused by EDC exposure in wildlife
OBSERVED EFFECTS OF EDCs IN WILDLIFE
Altered hormone levels
Brain and neurological problems
Changes in bone density and structure
Deformities in body and/or reproductive organs
Embryo mortality
Feminization of males
Impaired sexual behaviors
Impairment of thyroid function
Intersex
Masculinization of females
Modified immune system
Reduced fertility
Reproductive tissue cancers
Skewed sex ratios

2.1.1 Reproductive Toxicity of EDCs in Wildlife

In wildlife, depending upon the species, the age of exposure, and the specific EDC, exposure has been shown to result in altered reproductive function including:

- Masculinization: a process by which a female acquires male-typical traits.
- Feminization: a process by which a male acquires female-typical traits.
- Demasculinization: a process by which a male loses male-typical traits.
- Defeminization: a process by which a female loses female-typical traits.

Examples of reproductive aberrations caused by EDCs are summarized (Table 6). As an example of EDC masculinizing effects, female snails and mollusks should not develop a penis. However, some of these invertebrates developed male genitalia following exposure to a biocide contained in anti-fouling paint used to remove barnacles from boats and ships. Indeed, masculinization of marine gastropods exposed to tributyltin (TBT) has resulted in worldwide population decline and provides a definitive example in invertebrates of an endocrine-mediated adverse effect caused by EDC exposure. Although the exact endocrine mechanism is not yet fully understood, several hypotheses have been proposed including elevated androgen levels, alterations in aromatase activity (which converts androgens to estrogens), and modulation of the retinoid X receptor (RXR).

A number of studies have shown that exposure of fish to chemical components of pulp and paper mill effluents and sewage treatment effluents can result in disruptions of reproductive development and endocrine function. For example, male fish can be feminized by acquiring female-typical reproductive traits. Males can also be demasculinized, referring to a loss of the male phenotype. For instance, under normal circumstances, female fish respond to endogenous estrogen exposure by producing an egg yolk protein known as vitellogenin. Males also produce vitellogenin in response to estrogen, but because their normal levels of circulating estrogen are magnitudes of order lower than females, they usually have no detectable vitellogenin when assayed for this endpoint. However, male fish with feminized characteristics (higher estrogen levels, production of vitellogenin, an egg yolk protein) have changes to their gonads including the presence of ova within the testes. This was first reported for fish that were found downstream from sewage treatment outlets in England (Jobling and Sumpter, 1993) later found to have high concentrations of estrogenic substances. Although several mechanisms have been identified (i.e., alteration of sex steroid biosynthesis, agonism/antagonism of hormone receptor), the exact causative chemicals are controversial.

The detrimental reproductive effects of EDCs in turtles and alligators are well documented. For example, a marked population decline in alligators over the decade following a pesticide spill in Lake Apopka (FL, USA) is attributed to high levels of endocrine-disrupting organochlorine contaminants. Researchers found that chemicals from the spill were not only lethal to developing eggs but also altered sexual development of young animals (Guillette et al., 1994). Male alligators from Lake Apopka had decreased penis size, sometimes making them physically incapable of mating. In a follow-up study, the same chemical components measured in Lake Apopka alligator eggs were applied to turtle eggs in a laboratory experiment. In turtles, sex determination is controlled by temperature and is modulated by the presence/absence of estrogens and androgens. In exposed animals, investigators found that sex determination was shifted in a female direction by these compounds, demonstrating feminizing estrogenic effects of these EDCs (Willingham and Crews, 1999).

Starting in the 1950s, predatory and fish-eating birds faced a whole host of health issues, including poor reproductive success, as a result of organochlorine exposure. In birds exposed to DDE, a metabolite (breakdown chemical) of DDT, eggshell thinning, and abnormal gonadal development have resulted in dramatic population declines. Fish-eating birds exposed to PCBs through contaminated fish have developed GLEMEDS, a syndrome of embryonic abnormalities. Following a ban of DDT and PCBs in the USA, populations of bald eagles, brown pelicans, and other birds of prey began to recover. However, since organochlorine chemicals are persistent in the environment and still used for insect control in less developed countries, birds remain at risk.

The examples highlighted in this section provide clear evidence that EDC exposure has occurred in wildlife species across taxa. While the majority of compelling data for exposure come from organisms living in a highly contaminated habitat, there is a paucity of exposure data for low-level and non-persistent EDCs. However, considering that the mechanisms for reproductive toxicity in wildlife are virtually identical to those in laboratory animals—and these latter species are vulnerable to low-level exposures—we believe that low-dose effects of EDCs in wildlife have long-term detrimental consequences.

2.2   EDCs AND HUMANS

In humans, most of the studies on effects of EDCs have been conducted on highly exposed groups from accidental exposures or certain industrial occupations. Biomonitoring studies also show that humans are exposed to a complex mixture of known EDCs at levels typically on the order of parts per trillion (ppt). Although the available data raise concerns, evidence of direct causal association between low-level EDC exposure and adverse health effects is generally lacking, particularly for exposure during critical developmental periods that affect adult function. This is because the long life of humans, and lack of information about what, when, and how much exposures we each have had, makes causal relationships impossible to draw. Each person has a unique exposure pattern to known and unknown EDCs, and differences in body composition and metabolism contribute to a high variability between individuals. Nevertheless, EDC exposure is proposed to contribute to adverse health outcomes in humans (Table 7). Several examples of known exposures strengthen the evidence for human susceptibility to EDCs.

TABLE 7: Suspected EDC effects in humans
MALES
Cryptochordism—congenital malformation resulting in non-descended testes in male babies
Hypospadias—congenital malformation whereby the urethral opening is located on the underside of the penis, rather than at the tip of the glans penis, reduced semen quality
Testicular germ cell cancers
Prostate cancer
Timing of puberty (delayed or accelerated, depending upon EDC)
FEMALES
Precocious (early) puberty
Reduced fertility, fecundity
Polycystic ovarian syndrome (PCOS)
Change in sex ratio of offspring (fewer males)
Endometriosis
Uterine fibroids
Hormonal cancers
BOTH MALES AND FEMALES
Deficits in cognition, learning, and memory
Neurodevelopmental disorders such as autism, attention deficit disorder, mental retardation, cerebral palsy
Significant IQ deficits
Altered play behavior, aggression

2.2.1 Diethylstilbestrol (DES)

The most compelling example of human exposure to a hormone disruptor is provided by the story of the powerful estrogenic pharmaceutical DES. Millions of pregnant women in the US were prescribed DES to prevent miscarriage—and ironically, DES turned out to be ineffective in its intended use. Instead, DES exposure of the fetuses caused changes to their developing reproductive tract that often were not apparent at birth. Instead, women presented with reproductive tract abnormalities that came to light later in life and were linked to subfertility, infertility, or development of a rare form of vaginocervical carcinoma (Herbst et al., 1971). Male offspring had higher incidences of cryptorchidism (undescended testes). This was one of the few examples of the cause and effect of prenatal exposure to estrogenic hormones. In addition, and of great importance to the field of endocrine disruption, the timing of DES exposure (fetal) was associated with the latent development of disease in humans. These concepts will be elaborated upon in Chapters 3 and 4. Also, as will be discussed later (Chapter 6), there may be multigenerational effects on exposures as measured in the DES grandchildren. As a whole, the DES story, while unfortunate, has led to a much greater understanding of the vulnerability of the fetus, the potential for EDCs to have latent effects not seen for years or decades, and the propensity for effects to last for generations.

2.2.2 PCBs

There are two reported incidents of high-dose PCB exposure to humans via contaminated cooking oil [reviewed in (Quinn et al., 2011)]. The first, in 1968 in Japan, resulted in about 2000 people becoming ill from rice oil (Yusho) and the second in Taiwan in 1979 (Yucheng) are now case studies for effects of high-dose PCB exposures. In the adults who consumed the oil, there were symptoms of organochlorine poisoning, such as chloracne, ocular symptoms (lesions, discharge, eyesight changes), and pigmentation changes to skin. In exposed adults, there was an association between exposure and mortality from liver and respiratory cancer. Endocrine-disrupting symptoms were also seen, including irregular menstrual cycles, alterations in immune and respiratory function, and suspected changes to testosterone metabolism (Aoki, 2001).

Again, developmental exposure of children had adverse effects, especially on neurodevelopment. PCB exposures to young children impaired cognitive development including motor skills and IQ (Quinn et al., 2011). As studied in more detail in the Yucheng (Taiwanese) episode, exposure of fetuses and infants (via *in utero* and lactational exposure, respectively) was associated with poor cognitive development and delayed puberty in males (Aoki, 2001).

Since that time, other studies have indicated links between PCBs and related organohalogens with human disease. For example, consumption of contaminated fish from Lake Michigan by pregnant women was associated with neurocognitive impairments in the children (Jacobson and Jacobson, 1996). Studies of other cohorts around the world have confirmed such relationships (Grandjean and Landrigan, 2006).

2.2.3 Dioxins

In 1976, a chemical plant in Seveso Italy exploded, leading to the release of high levels of dioxins into the environment. Humans exposed to dioxins at various levels, depending upon how close they were to plant and wind currents, experienced a range of symptoms from overt poisoning by the major dioxin, TCDD, the most potent being chloracne, peripheral nervous system neuropathy, and elevated liver enzymes [reviewed in (Pesatori et al., 2003)]. The exposed population and their offspring have been carefully followed since that time for evidence of endocrine disruption, development of cancers, other phenotypic changes, and mortality. Some of the strongest correlations between TCDD concentrations in the serum were found for breast cancer risk, menstrual cycle abnormalities, and endometriosis in the adult women. While overall mortality over the next 20 years did not differ among groups, there was greater mortality in men for rectal and lung cancer and in both sexes for lymphatic and hemopoietic neoplasms, especially leukemia and multiple myeloma. Men had increased heart disease, and females had increased diabetes and respiratory mortality. Of great interest, and probably relevant to the endocrine-disrupting actions of dioxins, the birth ratio of children from parents exposed to the highest concentrations of TCDD was highly female-biased (Pesatori et al., 2003).

2.2.4 Low-Dose Human Exposures: What Is the Evidence?

The examples provided above are the best cause-and-effect evidence for EDC actions in humans. With the exception of DES, however, many of these effects of PCBs and dioxins are due to acute neurotoxicological actions. Thus, the question remains whether and how low-dose EDCs affect humans. In the past 5 years, several converging bodies of evidence have provided the strongest support to date that such effects are highly relevant. This work has been summarized in several important reports since 2007 on the subject (Box 1). Each of these studies provided a thorough and careful literature review on laboratory animal research, human exposures, epidemiological data, and drew conclusions that the weight of evidence supports concern for humans. Furthermore, the high conservation of endocrine and neurobiological processes in humans and animals provides very high certainty that laboratory animal studies reflect similar processes in humans.

The other issue of relevance to proving human exposures is the growing information about body burdens, assessed through biomonitoring (Calafat and Needham, 2007). The NHANES (National Health and Nutrition Examination Survey) database established by the CDC was started

---

Box 1: Landmark studies on links between EDCs and human health

- Faroes Statement on EDCs and human health concerns: (Grandjean et al., 2007).
- Chapel Hill Consensus Statement on BPA: (vom Saal et al., 2007).
- Endocrine Society Scientific Statement on EDCs: (Diamanti-Kandarakis et al., 2009).
- Review of low-dose EDC effects: (Vandenberg et al., 2012).

---

in the 1960s and continues to this date [http://www.cdc.gov/nchs/nhanes/about_nhanes.htm]. It includes demographic, socioeconomic, dietary, and health and medical information on participants. An arm of NHANES on environmental exposures is relevant to understanding EDCs and humans. The most recent (4th) report on Human Exposures to Environmental Chemicals was published in 2009 based on data collected from 1999 to 2004 on exposures to 212 chemicals. Its goal was to provide estimates of exposure in the US population, to establish reference values, to determine whether there are population differences, and to inform future research and priorities. Results of NHANES included the presence of a polybrominated diphenyl ether, BDE-47, in serum of nearly all sampled individuals. BPA was found in urine of more than 90% of samples. Perfluorinated chemicals (e.g., PFOA) also had widespread detection. These datasets have been used as a launching point for subsequent research. For example, the NHANES dataset was used to draw the conclusion that half-life of BPA was longer than originally predicted(Stahlhut et al., 2009). A limitation of NHANES is that it is cross-sectional (i.e., it does not include longitudinal data). It also does not take developmental exposure into consideration; as articulated by the authors of a review chapter, "Therefore, a pressing need exists for assessing exposure during critical periods of development—a period of increased susceptibility to the potential adverse effects of EDCs" (Calafat and Needham, 2007). The German Environmental Surveys (GerESs) has conducted large-scale surveys of exposure to environmental chemicals [reviewed in (Calafat and Needham, 2007)]. This program is important because it is beginning to study children from 3 to 5 years of age.

2.3   SUMMARY AND CONCLUSIONS

There are numerous chemicals in our environment with endocrine active properties, and these are routinely detected in human, wildlife, and environmental (i.e., soil, air, water) samples. Some of these EDCs are persistent, while others are not. Some are lipophilic, concentrating in the body's fat stores and secreted in milk, while water-soluble EDCs may only be present for short periods of time but at critical developmental stages. We are just beginning to appreciate the magnitude of

human and wildlife EDC exposure, and the consequences on health and disease. Human susceptibility to EDCs is perhaps best demonstrated by examples of highly exposed groups from accidental
exposures to compounds such as PCBs or dioxins. While these unfortunate incidents provide the
most compelling evidence of a direct causal association between EDC exposure and adverse health
effects, the impact of low-dose exposures during critical developmental periods has not yet been
adequately studied. Future research assessing exposure during these periods of marked vulnerability
will undoubtedly helps clarify the cause-and-effect relationship between EDC exposure and human
health outcomes.

.   .   .   .

CHAPTER 3

EDCs and Development

3.1 VULNERABILITY OF THE DEVELOPING FETUS

The concept of environmental endocrine disruption is inextricably linked to development. Normal prenatal and early postnatal development are life stages during which the body undergoes enormous change. Waves of gene activation and repression are responsible for the normal patterning and development that occurs in the body and brain. Obviously, an individual's genes contribute an enormous amount to these developmental processes. In addition, the environment can interact with these genes to modulate their expression.

In the case of a mammalian fetus, the placenta and amniotic fluid form the immediate environment and provide nutrients and remove waste products. The placenta and amniotic fluid also are a source of hormonal exposures to the fetus as the placenta is an endocrine organ. Both maternal and fetal hormones change prenatally and are critical for normal fetal development. Fifty years ago, it was thought that the fetus was protected from any potentially toxic compounds to which the mother came into contact. However, we now know that the placenta is not impermeable, and some chemicals can be transferred from mother to fetus. An excellent, although again unfortunate, example is provided by thalidomide—women who were prescribed with this drug to treat morning sickness often gave birth to babies with severe malformations. Another example, discussed in the previous chapter, is diethylstilbestrol (DES), used to avert miscarriage. Offspring developed reproductive tract malformations and in some cases, rare forms of cancer in early adulthood. Again, this highlights the transfer of chemicals across the placenta. When these chemicals act as hormones, or perturb the normal hormonal milieu of the fetus, as happened with DES and as is happening now with EDCs, this can affect fetal development—and permanently change the developmental trajectory of that individual. This can alter the propensity to develop a disease or dysfunction later in life, a concept referred to as the "Fetal basis of adult disease" or the "Developmental origins of health and disease" (Barker, 2003).

3.2 FETAL (DEVELOPMENTAL) BASIS OF ADULT DISEASE

The effects of EDC exposure largely depend on the period of life during which an organism is exposed. Gestation and infancy are developmental periods characterized by marked susceptibility to the effects of environmental toxicants. For instance, evidence from laboratory animals and epidemiological data from humans suggests that the risk of developing certain chronic diseases (including endocrine and neurobiological dysfunctions) during adulthood may be increased by exposure to certain EDCs during early life. The term "fetal basis of adult disease" refers to observations that the maternal environment during gestation and external environment of a developing organism interact with an individual's genes to determine predisposition to disease or dysfunction during adulthood or aging (Barker, 2003). As implied by the name, the consequences of developmental exposure may not be evident during early life, but may be manifested following a significant period of latency. For humans and other animals, reproductive function, a process that involves both neural and endocrine regulatory processes, is particularly sensitive to disruption by EDC exposure during early life due to rapid structural and functional changes that occur during the developmental processes of sexual differentiation and brain development.

3.3   CRITICAL DEVELOPMENTAL PERIODS

There are several developmental periods during which exposures to EDCs are most detrimental. Early fetal development is associated with not only sex determination but also with developmental changes to the germline (cells that become sperm or ova) that occur exclusively during this period. In the fetus, failure to be exposed to appropriate levels of natural hormones, or exposures to exogenous hormonally active substances, such as EDCs, affect genomic characteristics of the germ cells—and thereby affect not only the exposed fetus (F1 generation) but also the F2 generation which will develop from the F1's germ cells. Researchers are beginning to be concerned about transgenerational effects of EDCs—in other words, effects that are transmitted from generation to generation—and multigenerational studies are revealing consequences of fetal exposure that are perpetuated in this manner (Walker and Gore, 2011).

The perinatal period—late gestation and early postnatal life—is also a critical period in mammals. As will be discussed in more detail later, neuroendocrinologists have known for decades that the development of the brain is highly sensitive to steroid hormone exposures that occur shortly before or after the time of birth. In rodents, the male embryonic testis produces high levels of testosterone. Exposure of the brain to this hormone, as well as to testosterone's metabolite estradiol within nerve cells, is responsible for brain masculinization. (It may seem counterintuitive that estradiol masculinizes the brain, but this is indeed the case in rodents.) In primates, sexual differentiation is probably more strongly driven by testosterone as opposed to estrogen, but the concept of a critical period still applies. As a consequence of these differential prenatal hormonal exposures, the brains of males and females develop differently. These effects are manifested by differences in reproductive physiology and behavior that can be seen in adulthood and also include non-reproductive functions controlled by the brain. This late gestational period is a time when organisms are probably most responsive to EDCs. A large body of evidence shows that gestational EDC exposures permanently change the developing organism. As a result, the brain and behaviors differ later in life. In addition, propensities to develop hormone-sensitive cancers, metabolic dysfunctions, type 2 diabetes, and other endocrine disorders are increased by developmental EDC exposures. As a whole, this field of research and clinical practice relates back to the concept of the fetal (or developmental) basis of adult disease and dysfunction (Barker, 2003) discussed in the previous section. In other words, what an individual is exposed to as fetuses or developing infants could predispose for diseases later in life.

Other life stages are vulnerable to exposures, although possibly less so than early development. Throughout the life cycle, endogenous levels of hormones, and sensitivity to those hormones, undergoes fluctuations. For example, puberty, reproductive cycles (e.g., menstrual cycles in women), and aging (e.g., menopause) are life stages that exhibit large hormonal change. Thus, no life stage is immune to the potential effects of EDCs.

3.4   KEY TOXICOLOGICAL PRINCIPLES RELEVANT TO DEVELOPMENTAL EXPOSURES

There are several general principles utilized by toxicologists to understand the effects of chemicals on biological processes and to assess risk associated with exposure (Box 2).

Box 2. Considerations in assessing exposures

- Dose: How much chemical has the individual been exposed to?
- Duration: How long was the exposure? Was it acute or chronic?
- Age at exposure: Fetus, infant, child, adult—or lifelong?
- Nature: Which EDC—single compounds or mixtures?
- Response: The resulting biological effect.

A brief description of important toxicological principles as they pertain to developmental EDC exposures is provided below.

3.4.1 LOAEL/NOAEL

For decades, regulatory toxicologists have relied upon the assumption that for every chemical, there is a level of exposure at which there is no statistically significant increase in the frequency of adverse effects (alteration of morphology, growth, development, function or life span, etc.) in the exposed population compared to its unexposed control counterparts—a concept referred to as the *no observable adverse effect level* or NOAEL. The lowest observed adverse effect level (LOAEL) is the lowest dose at which there is an observed adverse effect. Toxicologists derive the NOAEL and LOAEL by testing the effects of high doses and subsequently reducing the dose until a level is reached at which no adverse effects are observed. Uncertainty factors are used to translate the LOAEL dose obtained from laboratory animals into a tolerable dose for humans, which is generally determined by dividing the LOAEL by 1000. For example, an uncertainty factor of 10 takes into account human variability, a further 10 is intended to allow for differences in metabolism, and 10 more for genetic susceptibility or a vulnerability, such as pregnancy.

The concepts of NOAEL and LOAEL are contingent upon the expectation that there is a "safe" dose. Biologists, especially endocrinologists, interested in hormone principles, understand that any exposure—no matter how low—may cause detrimental effects. In other words, there is no NOAEL or LOAEL in understanding effects of exposures to EDCs, and there is no "safe" dose (Sheehan, 2006). This concept is illustrated by thinking about developmental exposures. There are developmental stages at which a cell, tissue, or organism may have no exposure to an endogenous chemical to which it will be exposed at other life stages. Gonadal steroid hormones, such as estrogens and androgens, fluctuate greatly throughout the life stage, and there are developmental timepoints when the body is completely unexposed to these hormones. If one considers exposure to an exogenous EDC during one of these normally unexposed life phases, this would result in some change in the target cell (e.g., binding to a receptor; intracellular signaling; DNA modification) that could change the developmental trajectory of that cell (Vandenberg et al., 2012).

3.4.2 Dose–Response Principles and Why they Do Not Apply to EDCs

In toxicology, a dose–response relationship describes the change in a chemical's effect on an organism caused by different levels of exposure (doses) after a certain amount of time (duration of exposure). Often, the greater the dose, the greater the response (i.e., a linear relationship). This results in a simple monotonic dose–response curve, with low doses having small effects and high doses having big effects. We now know that this is a gross oversimplification when thinking about hormones and EDCs. In evaluating effects of EDCs on a particular endpoint, a very low dose of a hormone (or EDC) can have a potent effect; an intermediate dose a lesser effect; and a high dose a potent effect. This results in a U-shaped dose–response curve, something that is seen frequently in physiological systems. Other dose–response curves may be inverted U in shape or have zig-zag patterns or shapes that are non-linear (Figure 5) (Vandenberg et al., 2012). In fact, recent commentaries on the relationship between EDCs and dose–responses have led to the conclusion that unlike in standard toxicological testing where "the dose makes the poison" in considering EDC effects, it is often "the timing that makes the poison."

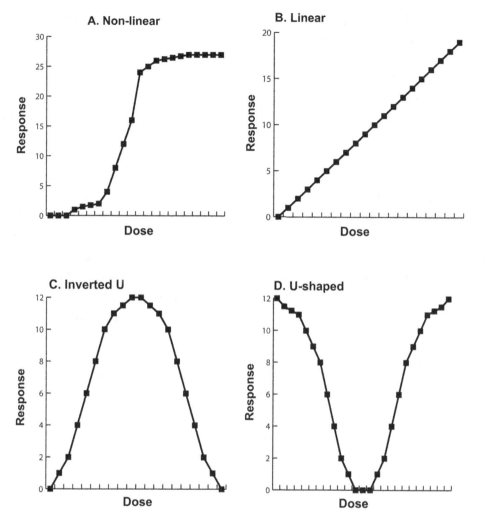

FIGURE 5: Representative dose–response curves seen in EDC research.

3.4.3   Low-Dose Effects of EDCs—Lack of a Threshold

Regulatory agencies have been relying upon the idea that health effects that do not occur at moderate or high levels of exposure to a compound cannot be induced by much lower exposure levels. However, a number of recent studies with EDCs challenge the premise of this traditional regulatory concept and demonstrate that low-dose effects of EDCs are often quite different from high-dose effects and therefore cannot be accurately predicted from high-dose testing.

As discussed above, dose–response testing on hormone or endocrine disruptor effects often shows non-monotonic dose–response curves. Inherent in this principle is that sometimes very low doses have potent effects that are often not predicted by higher-dose testing. Indeed, as best exemplified by the estrogenic compound bisphenol A (**BPA**), extraordinarily low doses can have profound effects. This result, while counterintuitive, has held true again and again in biology. One explanation for very low-dose effects of EDCs is the differential sensitivity of an organism to exogenous substances depending upon the life stage. Early development (e.g., fetal, infancy) is a critical period of life when sensitivity to very low doses of EDCs may be the most devastating. Beyond development, though, is the concept that because the body is extremely sensitive to endogenous hormones, which can fluctuate widely under normal conditions in order to maintain homeostasis or to respond to the environment, we have evolved the ability to respond to a range of hormones, from very low to very high. Exogenous exposures, therefore, even at very low levels, can disrupt this homeostatic balance. Because these processes are biologically conserved, this concept applies to all organisms.

Concrete evidence for a lack of a threshold effect of EDCs was elegantly shown for a reptile model of sex determination (whether an organism develops into a male or a female). In mammals, sex determination occurs in the presence (male) or absence (female) of the SRY gene on the Y-chromosome. In many reptiles, including red-eared slider turtles, the same sexual differentiation pathways are triggered not by chromosomes but by temperature, with some temperatures favoring females and others favoring males. It is also known that in these reptiles, effects of temperature can be overcome by exposures to hormones during critical developmental periods when sex determination occurs. Work in this animal model has demonstrated the absence of a threshold in response to the steroid hormone, estradiol (Sheehan et al., 1999). This work translates to the absence of a NOAEL in toxicology testing. In addition, reptiles respond to estrogenic EDCs by a shift in the sex ratio towards female, showing that environmental estrogens, with no apparent threshold, can permanently alter the developmental trajectory.

We return to the case of bisphenol A (BPA), the additive used in many plastic products and food packaging. In mice, the estimated LOAEL is 50 mg/kg/day proposed by regulatory agencies (although we contend that LOAELs are not meaningful as discussed above). This translates to a "safe" tolerable daily intake (TDI) level for humans of 0.05 mg/kg/day (again, we disagree that there is such thing as a "safe" dose). Regulations are currently in place to ensure the general public is not exposed to levels of BPA higher than the TDI. However, the effectiveness of current safety regulations regarding EDCs has been called into question following a number of studies showing that BPA and other EDCs may show effects at levels orders of magnitude lower than the estimated LOAEL. This literature has been carefully reviewed recently, and we refer readers to (Vandenberg et al., 2012) for more details. Collectively, these studies show that low-dose effects cannot be reliably extrapolated from traditional high-dose testing. Very low levels of exposure, or even any exposure at all during critical developmental windows, may result in endocrine or reproductive abnormalities.

3.5   SUMMARY AND CONCLUSIONS

The developmental period between conception and infancy is particularly vulnerable to disruption by EDC exposure. In humans, the unfortunate examples of thalidomide and DES demonstrate that the effects of fetal exposure to exogenous chemicals may either be immediately evident at birth or remain undetected until adulthood. Moreover, results from recent multigenerational studies have prompted concern not only for the individual exposed during development but also their offspring due to transgenerational transmission of EDC effects. While early development appears to be the most sensitive to EDC disruption, other life stages characterized by large hormone fluctuation may also be impacted by exposure to EDC. In the last section of this chapter, we illustrated how traditional toxicological dose–response principles do not apply to EDCs. Indeed, as you will learn in greater detail in the following chapters, even exposure to minute doses of EDCs can disrupt development of brain regions that control cognition, reproduction, and behavior. Thus, for EDC exposure, regulatory toxicology cannot rely upon the premise that there exists a threshold dose below which no health effects are expected.

CHAPTER 4

EDCs and the Developing Brain

4.1   HORMONES AND BRAIN SEXUAL DIFFERENTIATION

Endogenous hormones produced by endocrine glands such as the gonad, adrenal, and thyroid, are critically important for normal brain development. Thus, perturbations of hormone actions by EDCs have substantial and wide-ranging consequences on neurobiological functions. We will begin this chapter by discussing how steroid hormones exert actions on the nervous system, focusing on developmental periods. Part of this discussion includes the topic of brain sexual differentiation, the process by which the developing brain develops physical and functional attributes that are manifested in adulthood as sex differences in behavior and neurobiological processes. The focus of this chapter will be on differentiation of the hypothalamus because this is the brain region most intimately connected to hormonal functions, including the neurobiology of reproduction. However, other brain regions are also hormone-sensitive and undergo developmental sexual differentiation, which will be discussed later.

Gonadal steroids are crucial for neural differentiation, survival, and phenotype, with developmental sex differences in levels of sex steroids leading to sex differences in brain structure and function. The topic of brain sexual differentiation is huge; we refer readers interested in this subject to another book in this series for further information as we cannot possibly cover all the nuances of this fascinating field (McCarthy, 2011). However, we will provide some general background to set the stage for understanding effects of EDCs on brain sexual differentiation, discussed later in this chapter.

Early life (fetal and infant) is a particularly important time when endogenous sex steroid hormones have what are referred to as "organizational" effects on the developing nervous system. Thus, sex differences in levels of, and exposures to, estrogens and androgens, affect neurobiological development in a sex-specific manner. These early life "organizational" effects of hormonal exposures are manifested later in life as sex differences in brain and behavior, a phenomenon that requires a second hit of hormones from the pubertal gonads. Puberty is considered to be a critical life stage for these "activating" effects of hormones; in addition, recent evidence indicates that further organizational effects of steroids can occur in concert with the activating effects at puberty (Sisk and Foster, 2004).

Sex differences in reproductive physiology and behavior are associated with phenotypic differences in the neuroanatomy and neurochemistry of specific brain regions. During critical developmental windows, especially perinatal development, there are sex differences in exposure of the brain to steroid hormones. As a consequence, differences in sizes of specific brain regions, numbers and morphology of cells, cellular phenotype of neurons (e.g., expression of receptors), and neurochemistry are established (McCarthy, 2011). In fact, these differences are in many cases permanent and can be measured across the lifespan.

A key component in the determining how a brain develops in a male- or female-typical pattern is the presence or absence of the testicular hormone testosterone and its aromatization to estradiol by the enzyme p450 aromatase. In rodents, the best-studied species, the male testis produces high levels of testosterone. This testosterone circulates in the fetus' body and can enter the brain. There, testosterone can bind to androgen receptors (ARs) and affect the target cells. In addition, many neurons express aromatase, which can convert testosterone into estradiol. This estrogen can bind to ERs in the brain. The combination of testosterone and estradiol in the male brain is critical for masculine brain sexual differentiation. Perturbations in this pattern (e.g., abnormally low exposure to androgens and/or estrogens) will feminize or demasculinize the male.

In female rodents, the ovary is relatively quiescent compared to the male testis. Thus, there is less gonadal hormone to begin with in the circulation. In addition, the steroid binding protein α-fetoprotein (AFP) forms a complex with any circulating endogenous estrogen, which prevents it from entering the brain (Bakker et al., 2006). Therefore, the low levels of estrogens produced by the female ovary are bound to AFP, making them unable to enter the brain. As a consequence, exposure of the female rodent brain to gonadal hormones is thought to be far lower than in males. These female-typical exposures to hormones (relatively low levels) are necessary for normal feminine brain differentiation. Aberrations in hormone exposures (e.g., increased levels of estradiol or testosterone) to females can masculinize or defeminize the female.

4.1.1 Hormones and Neuronal Survival and Death

Neuronal exposure to sex-appropriate levels of fetal hormones has potent effects on cell survival or death. It is known that apoptosis—or programmed cell death—is an important mechanism by which the brain develops. During fetal development, as neurons are born, connections are formed, and synapses are consolidated, some neurons are destined to survive and others to die. The process of apoptosis is highly sensitive to steroid hormones, and sex differences in estrogens and androgens result in profound differences in numbers of neurons, sizes of brain nuclei, and ultimately, brain functions (Forger, 2006) (Figure 6).

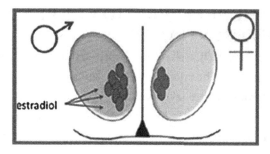

FIGURE 6: Representation of the sexually dimorphic nucleus of the preoptic area (SDN-POA) in the basal hypothalamus of adult male and female rats. The SDN-POA is initially similar in volume at birth, but neonatal testicular hormones (in this case estradiol, which is aromatized from testosterone within the brain) promote cell survival in males. By contrast, the female SDN-POA is much smaller due to apoptosis of neurons under conditions of very low ovarian hormone exposures. From McCarthy (2011).

In the SDN-POA, spinal nucleus of the bulbocavernosis, and bed nucleus of the stria terminalis, there are greater numbers of apoptotic cells in female than male rodents—and consequently, these regions are larger in males than in females later in life. By contrast, in the anteroventral periventricular nucleus (AVPV), which is larger in females than males, there is greater apoptosis in male rodents.

Developmental stage is critical in determining effects of hormones on neuronal apoptosis or survival (Rhees et al., 1990; Simerly, 2002). If neonatal females are exposed to testosterone or estradiol, their preoptic area is larger (masculinized) compared to an unexposed female. Conversely, castration of males neonatally results in a smaller, demasculinized (feminized) preoptic area. Similarly, the rat AVPV, which normally is larger in females, is sensitive to hormone influence during a period spanning late prenatal and early postnatal development (Patisaul et al., 2007). Thus, neonatal castration in males, or treatment of females with testosterone or estradiol, abolishes this sex difference in cell number and AVPV volume.

Sexual differentiation also involves developmental changes in the phenotype of neurons. This has been very well studied for the AVPV, which is dimorphic in expression of dopaminergic neurons, indicated by immunohistochemistry of the dopamine-synthesizing enzyme, tyrosine hydroxylase (Simerly, 1989). It is also dimorphic in kisspeptin expression (Kauffman et al., 2007) and ERα (Simerly et al., 1997). These neuronal phenotypic differences are established by pre- and perinatal hormone exposure, and perturbed by manipulations of perinatal hormone levels. As discussed below, exposure to EDCs at inappropriate times could cause permanent alterations in the differentiation of these developmental processes, with consequent changes in neuronal number, phenotype, and function.

4.2 EDCs AND THE PERTURBATION OF BRAIN SEXUAL DIFFERENTIATION

As discussed in earlier chapters, EDCs share many properties of endogenous steroid hormones. They bind (albeit weakly) to steroid hormone receptors, and they act on pathways that are involved in steroid signaling (e.g., steroidogenic enzymes such as p450 aromatase; co-factors and other transcriptional activators/repressors). They also have the propensity to bypass some of the body's protective mechanisms to limit exposure of the brain to hormones. For example, it is postulated that EDCs may not bind well to plasma binding proteins, including α-fetoprotein, which in other ways protects the female brain from exposure to circulating estrogens in early life. Thus, estrogenic EDCs may act in the developing fetal brain, even at very low levels (Vandenberg et al., 2012) to interfere with brain sexual differentiation.

There has been considerable recent research and interest in whether and how environmental EDCs perturb brain sexual differentiation (Gore, 2008). Research in the field has, in many ways, paralleled the basic research in hormones and brain sexual differentiation discussed in the previous section. For example, there is evidence that EDCs cause changes to neuronal survival/apoptosis, the size of sexually dimorphic nuclei, neuronal phenotype, and ultimately, functional outcomes. We will review the evidence for these effects of EDCs in the following sections.

4.2.1 Hypothalamic Morphology

Several EDC classes have been studied for their effects on the developmental sex differences in cell numbers and size of hypothalamic nuclei and the underlying apoptotic mechanisms caused by EDCs. Most research has focused on the AVPV and another subregion of the preoptic area—the sexually dimorphic nucleus of the POA (SDN-POA), so the focus of discussion will be these brain regions. As a whole, the literature on EDC exposures during perinatal life strongly supports the contention that exposure has permanent effects upon the developing hypothalamus, beginning with morphological changes and extending to disruptions in physiology and behavior.

Regarding the AVPV and SDN-POA, several classes of EDCs are known to change nuclear volume and cellular phenotype. To some extent, results have not always been consistent due to different EDC choices, timing of exposure, and sex and species differences, but overall there appear to be effects of neonatal EDCs on the morphology of sexually dimorphic brain regions. There is a relatively large literature on phytoestrogen effects, with numerous reports on developmental exposures to genistein and resveratrol and consequences on AVPV and SDN-POA volume. For example, maternal resveratrol consumption resulted in larger AVPV and smaller SDN-POA volumes in adult male rats, with no effect on these endpoints in females (Henry and Witt, 2006). By contrast, early postnatal exposure to genistein increased SDN-POA volume in female rats but had no effect in males (Lewis et al., 2003).

Similarly, organohalogens, such as dioxins, affect brain differentiation. Exposure to prenatal or early postnatal dioxins in rats decreased the SDN-POA volume in males (Ikeda et al., 2005) but had no effect in females, consistent with a demasculinizing effect. Other pharmaceutical estrogens, including DES and ethinyl estradiol, may have comparable effects (Gore, 2008).

4.2.2   Hypothalamic Developmental Apoptosis

As discussed earlier in this chapter, developmental apoptosis plays a very important role in determining the size and phenotype of sexually dimorphic brain nuclei. These apoptotic processes of cell survival and death are permanently altered by EDCs (Gore, 2008).

Effects of relatively few EDC classes on developmental apoptosis have been studied in the nervous system. Phytoestrogens have been reported to alter expression of apoptotic genes and to affect numbers of apoptotic neurons in male rats. In our own laboratory, we found that exposures of fetal rats to PCBs resulted in increased numbers of apoptotic cell numbers in the AVPV of female but not male rats (Dickerson et al., 2011a). As a consequence, we predict that the AVPV of female rats would be smaller—consistent with defeminization/masculinization caused by this endocrine disruptor. That study did not find any effect of PCBs in the medial preoptic area, showing the regional specificity of developmental exposures. To our knowledge, other studies have not directly related endocrine disruptor exposures to developmental apoptosis, but we believe that future results will show actions of these compounds on hypothalamic morphology.

4.2.3   Neuronal Phenotype

Many studies on how developmental EDCs affect neuronal phenotypic expression have focused on the estrogen receptors, particularly ERα, as experimental endpoints. We will briefly summarize the literature here and provide references for further information. Genistein exposure of neonatal rats decreased both the number and the percentage of cells in the AVPV that coexpressed tyrosine hydroxylase and ERα of female but not male rats (Patisaul et al., 2006). However, another study did not find an effect on gene expression of either ER in rats (Takagi et al., 2005), a difference that may be attributable to molecular (gene expression) vs. protein (co-expression of TH and ERα) in the studies. Bisphenol A, as an estrogenic EDC, is not surprisingly associated with developmental effects on differentiation of ER expression. Postnatal BPA exposure changed gene and protein expression of ERα in a dose- and developmental age-dependent manner (Aloisi et al., 2001; Monje et al., 2007).

Developmental PCB exposures affect hypothalamic differentiation, including gene and protein expression of the estrogen receptors. For instance, gestational exposure to A1254 (a commercial PCB mixture) increased ERα gene expression in the ventromedial nucleus of the hypothalamus (VMN), a region important for feminine sexual behavior, in female rat embryos (Lichtensteiger et al., 2003). Our own laboratory published recent data on how PCB exposure on embryonic days 16 and 18 (the third trimester in rats) affected expression of ERα immunoreactive cell numbers in the hypothalamus, specifically the AVPV. Although we did not find an effect of PCBs on this endpoint when rats were examined on postnatal day (P) 1 (Dickerson et al., 2011a), a significant decrease in ERα immunoreactive cell numbers was detectable on P60 (Dickerson et al., 2011b). In addition, an interesting outcome of that study was that whereas females had higher ERα cell numbers than males on P60 (consistent with the literature), prenatal PCB exposures caused this to be masculinized/defeminized (Figure 7).

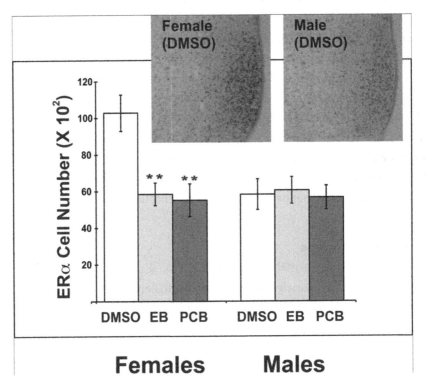

FIGURE 7: ERα immunoreactive cell numbers in the AVPV of male and female rats exposed gestationally to PCBs, estradiol benzoate (EB) or vehicle (DMSO) were counted in adult rats (P60) by unbiased stereological methods. Numbers of cells were higher in female than male vehicle-treated rats. Both PCBs and EB caused a significant decrease in ERα cell numbers in the females only, to levels similar to those in males. A representative micrograph of ERα expression in a control female and male is shown, with black dots indicative of immunolabel in cell nuclei. Modified from Dickerson et al. (2011b).

As a whole, this literature shows that early life EDC exposures cause developmental changes to brain sexual differentiation, a process that likely involves interference of normal hormone actions that are mediated by receptors in the brain and that affect neuronal cell survival or apoptosis.

4.3   EDCs AND REPRODUCTIVE BEHAVIORS

One of the most important consequences of developmental exposure of the brain to gonadal hormones is the organization of neural pathways that are involved in the sex-appropriate manifestation of reproductive behaviors. Sex differences in hypothalamic regional volumes and phenotypic differences in neurons are highly correlated with behaviors. In addition, reproductive behavior requires the activation of those neurobiological systems that were organized early in life. During puberty, the male and female gonads begin to secrete larger and larger amounts of sex steroid hormones, which can act on the adolescent brain. For example, pubertal hormones cause changes to neural circuits including neurite outgrowth, synaptic plasticity, and expression of molecules and receptors within or on neurons. These activational processes enable the brain to continue its postnatal development and ultimately to acquire the adult neural circuits that enable appropriate behaviors to be manifested.

Neonatal EDCs affect most of the same circuits, brain regions, pathways, and receptors involved in sexual behavior as do endogenous hormones. Mating behavior in rodents includes female-typical behaviors associated with proceptivity such as dart hopping and ear wiggling. These behaviors communicate to the male that the female is willing and able to engage in sexual activity. Once the mating process begins, females demonstrate their receptivity through a behavioral repertoire that includes the lordosis posture, in which the female arches her back and exposes her anogenital region for inspection and subsequent copulation. Males also engage in a stereotypical mating routine, beginning with mounting the female, followed by penile intromissions, and concluding with ejaculation.

Effects of EDCs on sexual behavior have been documented for many compounds and in numerous species. We begin with a discussion of effects of pre- or perinatal PCBs in rats. In female rats, Clemens' group has consistently shown that such PCB exposures perturb mating behaviors (Wang et al., 2002). Our group at the University of Texas at Austin examined effects of low-dose prenatal PCBs on paced mating behavior in the exposed females, tested in adulthood (Steinberg et al., 2007). We chose the paced mating protocol because it best enables a dissection of female-typical behaviors through enabling the female to choose whether, and at what pace, to mate (Erskine et al., 2004) (Figure 8). The most interesting results of our study were that females took more time to return to the male after an event (mount, intromission, or ejaculation) and that it took more mating trials for a female to show receptivity (Steinberg et al., 2007). Recent unpublished work in our lab, using a standard mating protocol (as opposed to paced mating) found fewer effects of prenatal PCBs, probably because under the "forced" mating conditions, the timing of most events cannot

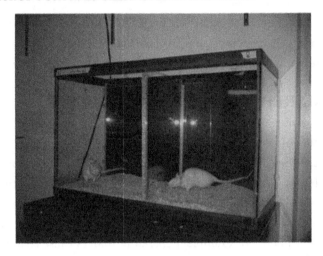

FIGURE 8: The paced mating arena is shown. A large aquarium is partitioned in half with a Plexiglas barricade. There are two small holes cut at the bottom of the barricade, small enough for the female to pass freely between the two sides of the aquarium. However, the male is too large to pass through the holes, confining him to one side. During the paced mating test, the female and male rats' behaviors are scored. Importantly, the amount of time that the female spends "pacing" the mating—that is, how much time she spends with the male, how often she leaves the male, and how long she spends away from or with the male, is scored for each behavioral event of mount, intromission, and ejaculation by the male.

be scored. Nevertheless, we found that females prenatally exposed to PCBs took longer to begin to engage in mating (Kermath et al., unpublished).

Detrimental effects of other EDCs on mating behavior of female rats have been reported. Phytoestrogens (e.g., soy) diminish lordosis behavior in female rats (Patisaul and Jefferson, 2010). Perinatal exposure to the pyrethroid insecticide fenvalerate also significantly reduced the lordosis quotient in female rats as adults (Moniz et al., 2005). The consequences of these studies are diminished reproductive success.

There are also published studies on effects of endocrine disruptors on reproductive behaviors in males. As in females, phytoestrogens given to developing male rats reduced the numbers of mounts and ejaculations and the latency to first mount and ejaculation (Whitten et al., 1995). Resveratrol exposure resulted in decreased mount frequencies in male rats (Henry and Witt, 2006). Other EDCs, including BPA, methoxychlor, and vinclozolin, are associated with diminished aspects of masculine mating behaviors in mice (Panzica et al., 2007).

The Japanese quail is a well-studied model for sexual behavior, as these animals are easily bred in captivity and are extremely well characterized for hormones and brain sexual differentiation [reviewed in (Panzica et al., 2007)]. It is also possible to apply EDCs directly to the eggs, unlike in mammals, where prenatal exposure requires treatment of the dam and potential confounds of maternal behavior. Experiments using quails have shown consistent adverse effects of low-dose EDCs, with outcomes ranging from embryonic mortality, postnatal morbidity, reproductive tract malformations, and other gross abnormalities. In addition, more subtle effects of less toxic doses were found on brain sexual differentiation and on sexual behavior. Genistein, DDE (a metabolite of DDT), vinclozolin (a fungicide), and methoxychlor (a pesticide) all caused decreases in aspects of male copulatory behavior (Panzica et al., 2007). As a whole, these studies on quail, taken together with published literature on rodents, suggests that sex differences in the nervous system induced by early life EDC exposure have long-lasting consequences on reproductive behaviors in adulthood.

4.4   EDCs AND NON-REPRODUCTIVE BEHAVIORS

While previous sections in this chapter have focused on the hypothalamus as a target of EDCs, the entire nervous system expresses hormone receptors in a developmental-, regional-, and sex-specific manner. Therefore, neurons in hippocampus, cortex, throughout the brainstem, and other regions, are potential EDC targets. In addition, neurons and glia that produce and release neurotransmitters, neuropeptides, and other neuroactive factors can be targeted by EDCs known to act directly on these molecules. For example, dopaminergic neurotransmission—including dopamine release, uptake, biosynthesis, and expression and function of dopamine receptors—are sensitive to certain EDCs such as PCBs (Seegal, 1996). In addition, EDCs can change neural properties such as those involved in synaptic transmission, signal transduction, membrane structure, receptor properties, and other characteristics.

The effects of EDCs on the brain are likely amplified during embryonic development, a time of maximal neuronal and behavioral plasticity. The development of normal neurobiological functions—and perturbations of these functions—comes about from a complex interplay of environment and genes. Endogenous hormones play key roles in sculpting these developmental processes, and as discussed earlier, gonadal steroid hormones are necessary for brain sexual differentiation. Thyroid hormones are necessary for appropriate neural growth, proliferation, and the euthyroid (normal) condition must be in place at birth to avoid significant cognitive dysfunction and mental retardation. Glucocorticoids near the time of birth are critical for the induction of labor.

What is less apparent is how developmental hormones affect non-reproductive behaviors. Much research has focused on behaviors related to cognition, learning, and memory, involving numerous brain regions including cortex, hippocampus, and amygdala. As we will discuss below, these brain regions, and the concomitant behaviors they control, are susceptible to endocrine disruption. Furthermore, these behaviors, while not directly related to reproduction, are still sexually dimorphic as they differ between males and females.

4.4.1 Hormones and Synaptic Plasticity

The synapse is a dynamic or "plastic" unit undergoing changes in structure and function in response to neural signals. The fact that there is considerable synaptic plasticity in the brain is not surprising when one considers cognitive processes such as learning and memory. We must be able to learn and remember in order to be able to adapt to our environment. Neuroplasticity and synaptogenesis are highly regulated by steroid hormones such as estrogens and androgens (McEwen et al., 1991). Sex differences in cognitive functions and learning and memory skills that are mediated by the hippocampus, cortex, and related brain areas are probably organized and activated in a similar manner to processes described for the hypothalamus above. In the following sections, we will focus on the role of the hippocampus, which plays a crucial role in cognition, learning, and memory (Bliss and Collingridge, 1993), and is well-studied for steroid-dependent neural plasticity (Hao et al., 2003).

Hippocampal synaptogenesis is strongly affected by endogenous and exogenous hormones. This structural plasticity caused by hormones is believed to underlie functional sex differences between men and women in behaviors such as spatial learning and memory controlled by the hippocampus (Sherwin and Henry, 2008). In women, there are also significant differences in performance of these tasks that vary across the menstrual cycle, before/after menopause, or after oophorectomy (surgical removal of the ovaries). Monkey and rat models show similar effects of hormones on cognitive processes, demonstrating the conservation of these actions.

4.4.2 EDCs and Neural Plasticity

Developmental EDC exposure has been linked to changes in neuroplasticity in general, and hippocampal plasticity in particular. The underlying mechanisms for effects of EDCs on synaptic plasticity involve the same molecular pathways described for steroid hormones above. A review of animal research on the subject (Schantz and Widholm, 2001) shows consistent links between EDCs and cognitive/behavioral outcomes, for a wide range of EDCs. In mice, tests of memory show that developmental exposure to BPA caused significant impairments in adulthood (Tian et al., 2010), a study that also showed that several neurotransmitter systems involved in the performance of these tasks (NMDA receptors, dopamine system) were impaired. Prenatal BPA exposure to mice resulted in changes in social behaviors in a sexually dimorphic manner (Wolstenholme et al., 2011). Also, polybrominated flame-retardants (PBDE) exposure changed the intracellular signaling molecules involved in mediation of steroid hormone actions, such as synaptic and axon-related proteins, ion channels, and many other molecules (Dingemans et al., 2011). This group also showed that long-term potentiation, a major feature of hippocampal neurons that is required for learning and memory, was disrupted by PBDEs. Similarly, pesticide exposures had adverse effects on fetal neurodevelopment and synaptic plasticity pathways (Connors et al., 2008). PCBs interfere with dendritic spine formation in the hippocampal CA1 region and cause cognitive behavioral changes in rats (Weiss, 2002; Lein et al., 2007; Colciago et al., 2009). Along with the compounds described above, other EDCs associated with cognitive change include plasticizers (phthalates), industrial compounds (dioxins), organochlorine and other classes of pesticides and herbicides (chlopyrifos, DDT, dieldrin, atrazine), and heavy metals (cadmium, mercury, lead). While heavy metals are known neurotoxicants, at low doses, they act upon hormone receptors (Dyer, 2007) and exert endocrine-disrupting effects.

There is also an excellent example of how adult exposure to BPA has substantial effects on neuroplasticity. Young adult ovariectomized female monkeys were treated for 4 weeks with a vehicle, estradiol, BPA, or estradiol plus BPA (administered at dosages below levels considered "safe" for humans; Leranth et al., 2008). Compared to vehicle-treated monkeys, estradiol-induced markers of synaptogenesis (spine synapses) in several subregions of the hippocampus, an effect that was obliterated in the BPA monkeys. That same lab also discovered an impairment of testosterone-induced synaptic plasticity in adult BPA-treated male rats (Hajszan and Leranth, 2010). These studies show that both developmental and adult BPA exposures cause change to neuronal properties, neuroplasticity, and behavior.

These data in animal models are highly applicable to humans. In fact, PCBs, which cause cognitive behavioral changes in rats, have been shown to interfere with human cognitive development (Grandjean and Landrigan, 2006). However, in general, while causal links between EDC exposures and cognitive processes in humans are difficult to draw due to the many variables among individuals in terms of timing of exposure, dose, mixtures, etc., there are strong correlative and epidemiological data. In addition, demographic data support the role of the environment on neurobehavioral disorders, frequencies of which are increasing. Cognitive and behavioral disorders (e.g., ADHD) and autism-spectrum disorders are on the rise, with predictions that the environment alone, or the interaction of the environment with genes, contributing to this rise. Furthermore, these disorders are sexually dimorphic, underscoring the importance of hormones in their etiology. In terms of cognitive functioning, individuals with the highest body burdens of EDCs have lower IQ scores and perform more poorly on tests of cognitive function (Grandjean and Landrigan, 2006).

4.4.3   EDC Effects on the Brain's Dopamine Neurons

EDCs have direct effects on the brain's neurotransmitters systems, of which dopamine neurons have been best-studied. Dopamine neurotransmission begins with synthesis of this monoaminergic peptide from the amino acid precursor tyrosine, within the presynaptic neuron. There, dopamine is packaged into secretory vesicles, which store the dopamine within the presynaptic cell. When the dopaminergic neuron is stimulated by depolarization, secretory vesicles fuse with the terminal membrane and release the neurotransmitter into the extracellular space in the synaptic cleft. At the target postsynaptic neurons, dopamine binds to its receptors to trigger a series of intracellular events involved in signal transduction. Neurotransmission is terminated by changes to the receptors (e.g., internalization and/or degradation), and/or dopamine is removed from the synaptic cleft by dopamine transporters found on local glial cells or other nearby neurons.

The brain has several distinct populations of dopamine neurons with unique projections to other brain regions. For example, dopamine neurons in the substantia nigra of the brain are important for motor activity. The brain's dopaminergic reward circuitry includes neurons in the hypothalamus, nucleus accumbens, ventral tegmental area, and other brain regions. In addition, dopamine neurons in the hypothalamus are involved in prolactin release from the anterior pituitary. The target cells for each dopamine populations have their own specific complement of dopamine receptors and transporters.

EDCs can disrupt dopaminergic systems in several different brain regions. Some of these effects harken back to our discussion earlier of brain sexual differentiation, as some populations of hypothalamic dopaminergic neurons are sexually differentiated, due to organizing effects of developmental estrogens and androgens (Simerly et al., 1997). More specifically, in the AVPV, there are much higher numbers of dopaminergic cells in female than male mice due to actions of estradiol on the ERα. Developmental exposure to EDCs such as BPA affects the sexual differentiation of numbers of dopaminergic neurons in the AVPV of mice and rats, showing relationships among EDCs and critical periods of development, hormones, and neurotransmitters.

Other dopaminergic neuronal populations are affected by EDCs, especially during developmental exposure. Rats exposed to BPA, phthalates, or nonylphenol early in life showed changes in dopamine transporters and receptors in the striatum and midbrain. Motor activity of these rats was also impaired, showing a functional consequence of dopaminergic neurotoxicity (Masuo et al., 2004). Developmental exposure to these EDCs caused hyperactivity in adulthood, an effect associated with changes to midbrain dopamine receptors (Ishido et al., 2005). BPA caused decreases in tyrosine hydroxylase, the rate-limiting enzyme in dopamine synthesis, in the substantia nigra, of female mice (Tando et al., 2007). PCBs are well-established dopamine neurotoxicants (Seegal, 1996; Jones and Miller, 2008).

4.5 SUMMARY AND CONCLUSIONS

Sexual differentiation of the hypothalamus, directed by the action of steroid hormones, is crucial for the development of sex-appropriate reproductive function and behavior. Exposure to EDCs at inappropriate times in laboratory animals has been shown to alter neuronal number, phenotype, and function with consequent disruption of adult reproductive physiology and behavior. In addition to reproductive function, development of non-reproductive endpoints such as motor activity, cognition, learning, and memory may also be disrupted by early EDC exposure. While a direct causal link between EDC exposure and deficits in cognitive function in humans is difficult to establish, existing data from epidemiological and animal studies do support the need to invoke the Precautionary principle to reduce/avoid exposure to any suspected EDCs during development.

·   ·   ·   ·

CHAPTER 5

EDCs and Neuroendocrine Systems

5.1   NEUROENDOCRINE SYSTEMS OF THE HYPOTHALAMUS

The brain is the body's first responder to the environment. Of an individual's three systems involved in communicating with her world (nervous, endocrine, and immune systems), the brain is able to respond most rapidly through synaptic transmission. A lesser-known role of the brain is its function as an endocrine organ. In other words, some neurons are capable of releasing chemical transmitters (hormones) directly into the bloodstream, a fundamental property of endocrine systems. The hypothalamus, located at the base of the brain (Figure 9), is the central neuroendocrine organ. A subset of hypothalamic neurons has the capacity to extend axons to a highly vascularized region at the base of the brain. This area, called the median eminence, contains a capillary bed that extends along the pituitary stalk and forms a second bed within the anterior pituitary itself. Thus, the median eminence is a tiny capillary system that enables communication between brain and pituitary,

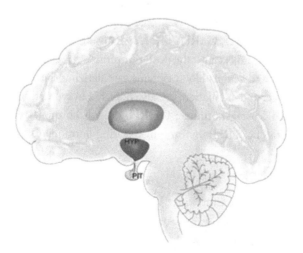

FIGURE 9: A sagittal view of the human brain is shown, with the front of the brain (anterior) on the left and the back of the brain (posterior) on the right. The hypothalamus at the base of the brain is depicted in blue, immediately above the pituitary stalk. Modified from Morrison et al. (2006).

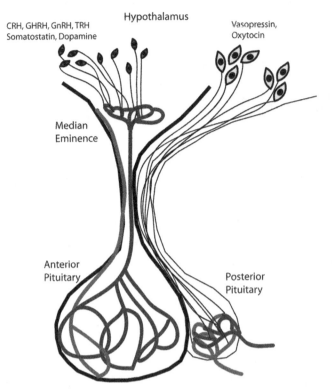

FIGURE 10: The hypothalamus is a neuroendocrine organ, releasing hormones into blood systems located between the hypothalamus and anterior pituitary, or from nerve terminals in the posterior pituitary directly into the general circulation. Neuronal populations in the hypothalamus that regulate the anterior pituitary (CRH, GHRH, GnRH, TRH, somatostatin, dopamine) are shown on the upper left. Neuronal populations that project into the posterior pituitary (vasopressin, oxytocin) are shown on the upper right. The arterial and venous blood systems vascularizing the anterior pituitary, and leading from posterior pituitary to general circulation, are also depicted in red and blue, respectively. Abbreviations: CRH: corticotropin-releasing hormone; GHRH: growth hormone-releasing hormone; GnRH: gonadotropin-releasing hormone; TRH: thyrotropin-releasing hormone.

and subserves the brain's endocrine functions (Yin and Gore, 2010) (Figure 10). Another subset of hypothalamic neurons, described below, projects their axons into the posterior pituitary, where the hypothalamic hormones are released directly into the general circulation—again consistent with endocrine function.

In most ways, hypothalamic neuroendocrine cells are just like other neurons: they express neural markers, they respond to synaptic input, they can be hyperpolarized or depolarized, and they have cell somata, axons, and dendrites. However, they differ from other neurons in that rather than releasing their signaling molecules at a synapse, they release them into the extracellular space in the vicinity of the blood vessels. Several hypothalamic hormones are referred to as hypothalamic releasing or inhibiting hormones. These hormones are responsible for the regulation of hormones in the anterior pituitary (Table 8). When the hypothalamic releasing or inhibiting hormones are transported to the pituitary via the portal capillary system, they act upon their receptors on specific pituitary target cells to regulate lactation, reproduction, basal metabolic rate, growth, and stress. Previously, the anterior pituitary was thought to be the body's "master gland," but it is now accepted that in order for the anterior pituitary to function, it must receive a hormonal signal from the appropriate hypothalamic releasing or inhibiting hormone. Thus, we now recognize the hypothalamus as the body's "master gland."

The hypothalamus also acts as an endocrine gland through its release of hormones from the posterior pituitary gland (Figure 10). In this case, hypothalamic neurons that synthesize vasopressin or oxytocin (primarily localized in the paraventricular nucleus and the supraoptic nucleus of the hypothalamus) extend axons into the posterior pituitary itself. The nerve terminals are abundant in secretory vesicles containing oxytocin or vasopressin. When stimulated by suckling (oxytocin) or changes in electrolyte balance in the blood system (vasopressin), the secretory vesicles in the posterior pituitary are released and gain access to blood vessels that transport these hormones through the general circulation. As is the case for the anterior pituitary hormones, the posterior pituitary hormones then circulate through the body, targeting receptors on specific organ systems such as breast, brain, and uterus (oxytocin) and kidney, blood vessels, and brain (vasopressin).

Endocrine and neuroendocrine systems serve an extremely important function: the maintenance of homeostasis in the body and the ability to adapt to environmental change. Imbalances in electrolytes and nutrients can result in illness or even death. Perturbations in energy balance are associated with the extremes of obesity and anorexia, or can cause behavioral changes. Endocrine systems respond to internal and external cues. For example, lactation is triggered by suckling of the infant at the mother's breast, a process that triggers the endocrine release of oxytocin and prolactin from hypothalamic neurons. Stress caused by external stimuli (e.g., a predator) triggers the release of glucocorticoids from the adrenal glands, a process that involves first the activation of central CRH hypothalamic neurons; their actions on pituitary cells that release ACTH; and finally the activation of the adrenal cortex glucocorticoids. Internal cues such as concentrations of glucose in the blood following a meal trigger the release of insulin and suppress the release of glucagon, in part through hypothalamic neurons that monitor and regulate energy balance. Thus, the endocrine and neuroendocrine systems serve as an interface between the organism and its environment.

As mentioned earlier, the endocrine system is one of the body's communication systems with the environment. It should be evident by now that the nervous and endocrine systems often work as

TABLE 8: Summary of the five neuroendocrine hypothalamic systems regulating anterior pituitary function

FUNCTION	HYPOTHALAMIC HORMONE(S)	ANTERIOR PITUITARY HORMONE(S)	TARGET HORMONE(S)
Stress	Corticotropin-releasing hormone (CRH): 41 amino acid peptide	Adrenocorticotropic hormone (ACTH), 39 amino acid peptide, encoded by POMC gene	Cortisol (humans) or corticosterone (rats, mice); steroid hormone family
Basal metabolism (thyroid)	Thyrotropin-releasing hormone (TRH): 3 amino acid peptide	Thyroid-stimulating hormone (TSH), composed of α and β subunits of ~100 amino acids each	Thyroid hormones (T3 and T4); lipophilic hormones synthesized from tyrosine and iodide
Growth	Growth-hormone releasing hormone (GHRH): 44 amino acid peptide Growth-hormone inhibiting hormone (GHIH, also called somatostatin)	Growth hormone (GH, also called somatotropin), 191 amino acid protein	Insulin-like growth factor-1 (IGF-1): 70 amino acid peptide
Reproduction	Gonadotropin-releasing hormone (GnRH)	Luteinizing hormone (LH), Follicle-stimulating hormone (FSH): they have a common α and a unique β subunit of ~100 amino acids each	Gonadal steroids (estrogens, progestins, androgens)
Lactation	Dopamine (prolactin-inhibiting hormone)	Prolactin (PRL): 198 amino acid protein	NA (milk is not a hormone within the lactating woman)

partners. As an example, consider a prey animal (a squirrel) spotting a predator (a fox). The squirrel must be able to detect the stimulus, something that happens within milliseconds through sensory processes transduced by the visual, auditory and olfactory systems via synaptic transmission. The nervous system also communicates to the endocrine systems. Through a series of efferents involved in sympathetic nervous system control, the adrenal medulla is stimulated to release adrenaline into the circulation. This rapid response initiates the "fight-or-flight" response in the squirrel, and also mobilizes energy stores and activates the cardiovascular system. At the same time, the stimulus of the fox is rapidly conveyed to the central endocrine systems in the brain. Specifically, neurons in the hypothalamus that produce the neuropeptide corticotropin-releasing hormone (CRH) are activated and release the CRH peptide into the blood system that vascularizes the pituitary. There, CRH binds to its receptors on a subset of pituitary cells, causing the rapid release of adrenocorticotropic hormone (ACTH) from the pituitary into the general circulation. At that point, ACTH is transported through the body, but its primary target is the adrenal cortex. The peripheral stress hormones, called glucocorticoids (cortisol or corticosterone) are released from the adrenal into circulation. Glucocorticoids mobilize glucose at the expense of protein and fat stores to enable the stress response to be maintained. This more prolonged endocrine response enables the squirrel to escape and recover.

This example underscores the point that there is a temporal progression in the ability of an organism to respond to its environment. First, the nervous system identifies and processes the predator through synaptic transmission. Second, the sympathetic nervous system is activated to trigger the endocrine release of adrenaline from adrenal medulla. Third, the hypothalamic (CRH)–pituitary (ACTH)–adrenal (glucocorticoid) axis becomes activated, a process involving three hormones and ultimately resulting in a more sustained response and adaptation of the body to a new homeostatic stress state, and ultimately, recovery from that state.

5.2   REPRODUCTIVE NEUROENDOCRINE SYSTEMS AND PERTURBATIONS BY EDCs

5.2.1   Background on GnRH Neurons

The control of reproduction begins not in the gonad or reproductive tract, but in the brain. In the hypothalamus, a population of about 1000 neurons synthesize and secrete the neuropeptide gonadotropin-releasing hormone (GnRH; Figure 11) into the portal vasculature leading to the anterior pituitary. There, GnRH binds to its receptor on cells called gonadotropes, which respond to GnRH with the synthesis and release of luteinizing hormone (LH) and/or follicle-stimulating hormone (FSH). From the anterior pituitary, these gonadotropins circulate through the body, targeting the gonads (ovary or testis). At the gonad, gonadotropins cause steroidogenesis (steroid synthesis) and gametogenesis (sperm production, ova production) and ovulation.

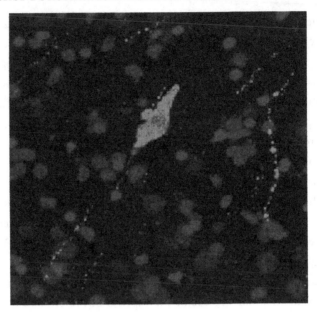

FIGURE 11: A photomicrograph of a representative GnRH neuron is shown, identified by immuno-label with a GnRH antibody. This neuron (green) can be seen in the basal hypothalamus of a rhesus monkey. As is typical of GnRH cells, the neuron appears to be ovoid in shape, with an axon projecting from the cell body to the lower left of the micrograph. Other GnRH processes can be seen as lines of green punctate labeling. Blue counterstaining (DAPI) shows other cell nuclei that are GnRH negative. For reference, the perikarya size is about 20 μm. (Courtesy Michelle Naugle and Andrea C. Gore.)

Although there are three levels of hypothalamic–pituitary–gonadal (HPG) regulation (Table 9), there is a hierarchical relationship. The top of the hierarchy is the hypothalamic GnRH neurons that provide the primary driving force on reproductive function. The GnRH peptide is stored in secretory vesicles within hypothalamic nerve terminals located at the base of the hypothalamus, called the median eminence (Yin and Gore, 2010). When stimulated, GnRH-containing neurons release this peptide into the extracellular space of the median eminence. From there, the peptide gains access to a capillary bed called the portal capillary system, which interconnects hypothalamus and anterior pituitary.

At the anterior pituitary, the GnRH peptide diffuses from the capillaries to its target cells, called gonadotropes. The gonadotrope cells synthesize/secrete the gonadotropins, LH and FSH. These cells express GnRH receptors on their cell surfaces, where GnRH binds to activate the intra-cellular signaling processes necessary for the synthesis of the gonadotropins. Upon stimulation, the gonadotropes quickly release the gonadotropins into blood vessels carrying these hormones into the

TABLE 9: Hypothalamic–pituitary–gonadal axis characteristics and hormones

TISSUE	CELL	HORMONE(S)	STRUCTURE
Hypothalamus (basal hypothalamus–humans; preoptic area and anterior hypothalamus rodents)	Neurons (~800–1000)	Gonadotropin-releasing hormone (GnRH) [also called luteinizing hormone–releasing hormone (LHRH)]	10-amino acid peptide, cleaved from a larger precursor
Anterior pituitary	Gonadotrope	Luteinizing hormone (LH) and Follicle-stimulating hormone (FSH)	There is a common α-subunit and unique β-subunit. LH's structure is α/LHβ, and FSH's structure is α/FSHβ
Gonad (ovary, testis)	Testis: Leydig and Sertoli cells Ovary: Granulosa and Theca cells	Sex steroid hormones: estrogens, progestins, androgens	Steroid hormones, derive from a cholesterol precursor following enzymatic actions (Figure 2)

general circulatory system. Although the gonadotropins are transported throughout the body, their primary targets are a subset of cells in the gonads, which express the LH and/or FSH receptors.

Within the ovary or testis, the gonadotropins act to regulate two major functions: gametogenesis (maturation of ova/sperm) and steroidogenesis (sex steroid hormone biosynthesis). With regard to steroidogenesis, the stimulation of target cells by LH/FSH causes a chain of enzymatic reactions, beginning with the cholesterol molecule and ending with one of the sex steroid hormones: progesterone, testosterone, or estradiol (see Figure 2 in chapter 1). All three of these classes of sex hormones are made in both males and females, but what differs between the sexes is the amount and the timing of their synthesis.

5.2.2 Sexual Differentiation of the HPG Axis

As discussed in Chapter 4, the brain is sexually differentiated due to a combination of genetic, hormonal and environmental factors. These sex differences extend to the control of reproductive physiology and behavior. In mammals, adults of both sexes release GnRH in a pulsatile manner, at intervals of about 30–120 minutes depending upon species. This type of intermittent GnRH release appears to be a critical property that is necessary to maintain reproductive function because constant GnRH exposure down-regulates the GnRH receptor on pituitary gonadotropes. There are some fundamental sex differences in GnRH pulsatility. Adult female rodents and humans experience reproductive cycles that vary in length in a species-dependent manner. For example, female rats have estrous cycles of 4–5 days, where female humans and many monkey species have menstrual cycles of approximately 28 days. Across the reproductive cycles, the frequency and amplitude of GnRH pulses changes, with larger amplitude pulses leading to the preovulatory GnRH/LH surge. By contrast, in males, GnRH pulses are not superimposed over a cyclic pattern of release.

A second and crucial sex difference in GnRH release relates to negative and positive feedback effects of steroid hormones. Males are under constant negative feedback regulation by testicular hormones. Thus, when testosterone (and probably estradiol) is high, this imparts information to the GnRH network to "turn down" the level of GnRH release. When testosterone concentrations are low, the negative feedback is relieved and GnRH neurons begin to "turn up" their release of the neurohormone from terminals in the median eminence.

In females, negative feedback prevails across most of the reproductive cycle. Thus, circulating estradiol levels tend to suppress hypothalamic GnRH, and pituitary LH/FSH release, for most days of the cycle. However, the period leading up to ovulation is characterized by a transition from negative to positive feedback. At this time in the cycle, the signal from rising peripheral estradiol becomes stimulatory, with higher estradiol levels driving higher GnRH and subsequently LH release. Ultimately, a GnRH/LH surge is initiated; the high levels of LH trigger ovulation (Kermath and Gore, 2012; Plant, 2012). It is suspected that there are probably species differences in these processes, with different relative contributions of hypothalamus vs. pituitary in positive feedback generation. Nevertheless, there is general agreement that a positive feedback signal from estradiol is unique to females and is a critical part of ovulatory functions.

Another sexual dimorphism in the control of GnRH neurons is the nature of the converging central nervous system inputs to the GnRH cells (see Figure 12 below). GnRH cells receive a large number of diverse signals from other neurons and glia. These inputs are similar in many ways between the sexes, but there seem to be some fundamental differences that relate to the unique ability of females to respond to positive feedback signals from gonadal steroids. Of particular note is the sexual dimorphism in afferent inputs to GnRH neurons from cells that synthesize and release the neuropeptide, kisspeptin. In rats, there are two populations of kisspeptin neurons, one in the AVPV and one in the arcuate nucleus (Kauffman et al., 2007). Sex differences in the neuroanatomy of these projections are organized by perinatal steroids. In addition, other neuroanatomical differences in the hypothalamus of males and females related to the GnRH neuronal network have been reported, and undoubtedly underlie sex differences in both pulsatile GnRH release and in steroid regulation.

5.2.3   Steroid Hormone Feedback and Regulation of HPG Function

The three levels of the HPG axis must function properly for reproductive function to occur normally. How then does the hypothalamus "know" how much GnRH to release to drive the rest of HPG function? Part of the answer to this question involves actions of circulating gonadal steroid hormones in the nervous system. Because steroid hormones derive from cholesterol—a lipophilic (fatty) molecule (Figure 2)—they are very small molecules with the ability to get across the blood-brain-barrier, and enter target cells by diffusion across lipophilic cell membranes. The brain is highly responsive to steroid hormones due to the high abundance of steroid hormone receptors, including estrogen receptors, progestin (progesterone) receptors, and androgen receptors in its tissues. The hypothalamus has particularly high abundance of these receptors (Simerly et al., 1990) and as a result, is very sensitive to feedback actions of steroid hormones.

Surprisingly, GnRH neurons themselves do not express most of the major steroid hormone receptors. So how do steroid hormones communicate their circulating levels to the HPG axis? This provides the rest of the answer to the question posed in the previous paragraph about how the hypothalamus "knows" how much GnRH to release. While GnRH neurons themselves do not express sex steroid receptors, they receive afferent synaptic inputs from other neural systems (Figure 12), many of which do express the gonadal steroid hormone receptors. It is now known that neurons that make synapses directly or indirectly upon GnRH neurons co-express estrogen, androgen and/or progestin receptors. These include many neuropeptide and neurotransmitter systems (kisspeptin,

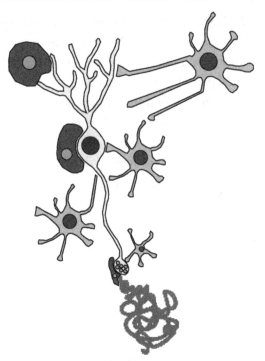

FIGURE 12: A complex network of neurons and glia makes inputs to a GnRH neuron (yellow). Multiple neurons (tan) make afferent inputs to GnRH cells at the level of their dendrites, cell bodies, and axons. In addition, several classes of glial cells (green) come into close contact with GnRH neurons at all of these levels. At the GnRH terminals, where the GnRH peptide is released into the portal capillary vasculature (red vessels), the glial cells that contact GnRH neurons are called tanycytes, and are involved in enabling GnRH neurons to have access to the portal vessels for their neurosecretory functions.

neuropeptide Y, norepinephrine, dopamine, acetylcholine, GABA, glutamate, vasopressin, oxytocin) and neurotrophic factors produced by neurons and glia such as the insulin-like growth factor (IGF) family and the transforming growth factor (TGF) family.

Thus, circulating steroid hormones are transported into the nervous system and act upon their target receptors on neurons and glia that converge upon GnRH neurons. Some of these inputs are excitatory and others are inhibitory to GnRH release; therefore, it is the overall sum of these parts that determines whether GnRH secretion is stimulated or inhibited. This point ties back to the fact that GnRH neurons are at the top of the hierarchy of the HPG axis controlling reproduction. Because GnRH neurons provide the final output from brain to pituitary and gonad, they may be envisioned as the base of a funnel channeling to pituitary. The middle of the funnel is all of the neurotransmitter/neurotrophic/neuropeptide inputs to the GnRH neurons, and at the top of the funnel are the steroid hormone signals mediated through these afferent intermediate neurons. The neck of the funnel is the GnRH nerve terminals that are projecting to the median eminence— the unique output of the hypothalamus in the control of reproduction (Gore, 2002). This means that GnRH neurons add up steroid sensitive signaling cues and turn this information into a "yes or no" decision about whether or not to cause GnRH peptide release.

5.2.4   Disruption of GnRH Neurons by EDCs

The sensitivity of GnRH neurons to endogenous hormone signals (albeit indirect) also means that this neuronal system is a likely target for environmental EDCs that may act upon steroid hormone receptors located on the neurons that make inputs to GnRH cells. The ability of GnRH cells to respond to the environment makes biological sense, because the reproductive HPG axis must be coordinated with environmental conditions to enable reproductive function to occur during times when the environment is right to facilitate reproductive success. Successful reproduction requires conditions that may not always be available in the wild such as the presence of a fertile opposite-sex mate, the availability of food and water resources, the appropriate season of the year such that offspring are born at a time when resources are abundant (e.g., the birth of spring lambs), and the absence of stressful or disease-promoting stimuli (e.g., predators or infections).

The evolution of the GnRH system to accommodate adaptation to the environment has also made the HPG system vulnerable to perturbation from environmental EDCs. Actions of EDCs on neurotransmitter systems that project to GnRH neurons, or to steroid hormones or steroidogenic enzymes in the brain that interconvert steroid hormones, can have downstream effects on GnRH regulation. Although there is still much to be learned about actions of EDCs on the GnRH system, the following sections provide evidence for GnRH neurons as targets for environmental EDCs.

5.2.4.1   *In vitro* Evidence.

GnRH neurons in the hypothalamus are not easily accessible for measurements of hormone release. They are widely scattered in the anterior hypothalamus and are few in number—only about 800–1000 GnRH cells can be detected in mammalian brains. As a result, it is difficult to study the properties of GnRH neurons in the living organism. In the 1980s, a team of researchers developed a mouse GnRH-secreting immortalized cell line—the GT1 cells—that can be grown in cell culture conditions and which have many properties of GnRH cells in the brain (Mellon et al., 1990). GT1 cells express the GnRH gene; they release the GnRH peptide at intervals of about 30 minutes—similar to the release patterns in mice; and they co-express many of the same receptors as GnRH neurons in the central nervous system. There are some differences between these cell lines and the brain, however. These cells have been reported to co-express steroid hormone receptors that are absent in GnRH neurons in animals. Thus, results on GT1 cells must be interpreted in line with these differences.

These GnRH GT1 cell lines have been used to study effects of several classes of EDCs: PCBs and organochlorine (methoxychlor, chlorpyrifos) and pyrethroid (tefluthrin) pesticides. Effects of the phytoestrogen, coumestrol, have also been published. We will discuss the results of these studies briefly, and we refer readers to a book chapter for experimental details (Dickerson et al., 2012). As a whole, this body of work shows that GnRH GT1 cells are sensitive to EDCs, suggesting direct neuroendocrine effects of these environmental contaminants. Our laboratory performed studies on effects of PCBs. Exposures of GT1 cells to PCB mixtures for 24 hours caused changes to the cellular morphology, release of GnRH, and GnRH gene expression. We also found neurotoxic effects of the PCBs and found a loss of cell viability due to a combination of necrotic and apoptotic mechanisms.

The organochlorine pesticides, chlorpyrifos and methoxychlor, were also tested for their effects on GT1 cells. Whereas GnRH peptide concentrations were unaffected, cellular growth and viability were changed. Chlorpyrifos caused cell proliferation and neurite extension, whereas methoxychlor was mildly neurotoxic. GnRH gene expression was stimulated by the pesticides at lower concentrations and inhibited at the highest concentrations.

The pyrethroid insecticide tefluthrin was tested on GT1 cell ion currents. Current amplitude and frequency were increased by tefluthrin. Finally, the phytoestrogen coumestrol was tested for its effects on GnRH gene expression in GT1 cells. Coumestrol had inhibitory effects on GnRH mRNA levels, effects that are at least partially mediated by the estrogen receptor ERβ.

Along with these studies on hypothalamic cell lines, EDC effects have been tested on GnRH neurons using *in vitro* cultures. Explanted hypothalamic dissections of 15-day old female rats were placed into a perifusion system. Parent, Bourguignon and colleagues studied how glutamate-evoked GnRH release, which happens reliably in these explanted hypothalami, was altered by several EDCs, particularly those in the dioxin family. They showed that o,p'-DDT had a large stimulatory effect on glutamate-induced GnRH secretion; BPA had a lesser effect (Rasier et al., 2008). Other EDCs such as p,p'-DDE and the pesticide methoxychlor had no effect in that study. These results show compound-specific effects of EDCs on properties of GnRH release from immature female rat hypothalamic explants.

Thus, *in vitro* work using GnRH cell lines and explants support the conclusion that environmental EDCs can directly target GnRH neurons.

5.2.4.2 *In vivo* Evidence.

The hypothalamic GnRH system is unique among central neuroendocrine systems. Developmentally, the hypophysiotropic GnRH system (that population of GnRH neurons that projects to the portal capillary vasculature to regulate pituitary gonadotropin release) originates embryonically from olfactory regions (Wray, 2010). A small population of these neurons, about 800–1000 total, migrates into the brain and targets the anterior hypothalamus and preoptic area. From there, the GnRH cell bodies extend an axonal process to the median eminence, where GnRH is released in pulses of about 0.5–1.5 hours, depending upon species. This anatomical organization is established shortly before birth. Disruptions of these processes by environmental EDC exposures prenatally could potentially affect this migratory pattern.

Because of their location at the base of the brain, their small numbers, and their scattered localization, it is difficult to measure GnRH release *in vivo*. Therefore, most of the research on effects of EDCs on GnRH systems has used GnRH gene expression (mRNA) as a more tractable endpoint. Other studies have measured gonadotropin levels in the circulation, especially LH, which can be detected from peripheral blood samples. Here, we will summarize the literature on effects of environmental EDCs on the GnRH systems of animals and provide evidence that the GnRH system is vulnerable to these factors.

5.2.4.3 Developmental EDC Exposures and GnRH Neurons.

Actions of EDCs on the GnRH system have been studied in a variety of vertebrate species including fish, birds, and mammals. Much of this research has focused on early life developmental exposure because the maturation of the GnRH system occurs in the embryo. Often, the outcome of effects on GnRH gene expression or hypothalamic–pituitary–gonadal physiology is measured later in life, especially in adulthood, because a developmental perturbation is not likely to be manifested until the age of reproductive competence has been attained. To follow is a discussion of evidence for developmental perturbation of GnRH neurons.

EDC studies on GnRH gene expression were conducted in ducklings whose mothers had consumed a plant phytoestrogen, daidzein, prior to conception. The ducklings, which had prenatal exposure as embryos, had decreased GnRH mRNA in their hypothalamus as young adults, and up-regulated GnRH mRNA after 1 year of age (Zhao et al., 2004). These results show that the age at which animals are evaluated is a critical factor, as effects of an early life endocrine disruptor exposure differs depending upon the life stage of the animal at the time of testing.

In rats, the literature on effects of developmental EDCs varies depending upon the nature of the EDC, the timing of exposure, and the endpoint of interest. We will provide a few illustrative examples. While maternal consumption of another phytoestrogen, genistein, did not affect GnRH gene expression in the postnatal rat pups (measured at 10 days of age) (Takagi et al., 2005), early postnatal exposure of rat pups (via lactational exposure from rat dams fed genistein) caused a decrease in GnRH gene activation, measured by co-expression of the immediate early gene product Fos in GnRH neurons of adult hormone-primed females (Bateman and Patisaul, 2008).

The estrogenic endocrine disruptor bisphenol A (BPA) was tested for its developmental effects on gonadotropin levels and on GnRH-induced LH release as assessed in adult female rats

(Fernandez et al., 2009). While basal LH levels and GnRH-stimulated LH release were reduced, GnRH pulses were increased, suggesting a change in pituitary responsiveness to GnRH caused by neonatal BPA. Another EDC study on BPA, together with the phytoestrogen genistein, reported that activation of GnRH neurons in adult females, evidenced by co-expression of the immediate early gene product Fos, was unaltered compared to vehicle-treated rats (Patisaul et al., 2007). Neonatal exposure of rats to PCBs, by contrast, resulted in a significant down-regulation of activated GnRH neurons [that co-expressed Fos; (Dickerson et al., 2011b)]. Finally, in rabbits, prenatal exposure to the fungicide vinclozolin decreased GnRH neuronal number (Bisenius et al., 2006), an effect accompanied by increased GnRH peptide and immunofluorescence in the median eminence, the site of GnRH terminals (Wadas et al., 2010). This latter result suggests that synthesis and/or transport of GnRH is altered in prenatally endocrine disrupted animals.

While these results may seem apparently contradictory, they suggest one general theme: In most cases, developmental exposure to EDCs causes changes to the GnRH system of laboratory animals. For the most part, the literature suggests that GnRH neurons are less active, evidenced by decreases (in some studies) in expression of the immediate early gene product Fos, by decreased GnRH peptide in nerve terminals, and diminished GnRH gene expression. These findings are also consistent with the work performed in slice explants of immature GnRH rats, showing diminished GnRH activation following glutamate stimulation. Finally, the work on GnRH cell lines suggests that at least some actions of EDCs on GnRH functional properties may occur directly on these neurons.

5.2.5 EDCs, Puberty, and the Brain

Puberty is the life transition during which an immature individual attains adult reproductive capacity. The pubertal process can be protracted, especially in long-lived species such as humans, where it takes several years. In rats, puberty requires about 2 weeks. In mammalian species studied to date, puberty begins with increases in GnRH pulse frequency and amplitude, followed by gonadotropin increases and ultimately, stimulation of sex steroid hormone synthesis and gametogenesis (sperm and egg development). Part of the pubertal process includes developmental changes in sensitivity to hormonal feedback. Research over the last few decades has conclusively shown that the brain drives the timing of the onset of puberty. The activation of GnRH is central to this process, as increases in pulsatile GnRH occur during puberty (Terasawa and Fernandez, 2001), but more importantly, exogenous stimulation of GnRH release accelerates the tempo of puberty.

Research on the central mechanisms driving puberty has concluded that the GnRH neurosecretory system is anatomically established by birth and that GnRH neurons have the capacity to release GnRH or to express the GnRH gene long before the timing of puberty. What is responsible for the acceleration of GnRH pulses and the increases in GnRH pulse amplitude that occur at puberty? Findings that GnRH neurons are regulated by afferent inputs from dozens of other neuronal and glial phenotypes explain this result (Figure 12). Neurotransmitters (glutamate, GABA, norepinephrine, dopamine, serotonin, and others), neuropeptides (kisspeptin, neuropeptide Y, neurokinin B, etc.), adipokines (leptin), neurotrophic factors (TGFs, IGFs), insulin, and energy balance regulators contribute to the regulation of the GnRH system. Of particular relevance to the timing of puberty, many of the neurons/glia that release these neuroactive substances are also steroid-sensitive. This is critical because GnRH neurons do not express most of the major steroid hormone receptors (estrogen receptor α, progesterone receptor, androgen receptor), and thus, feedback from these peripheral hormones must be mediated indirectly to GnRH neurons via afferent inputs. During puberty, there are developmental changes in regulatory inputs of GnRH neurons, the end result of which is to enhance GnRH neurosecretion.

5.2.5.1 Disruption of Puberty by Environmental EDCs.

Most research on endocrine disruption of puberty has been performed in laboratory rodents. In rats and mice, puberty is accompanied by secondary sex characteristic development, comparable to genitalia and breast development in humans. In rodents, the external markers of vaginal opening (an estrogen-mediated event), and preputial separation (an androgen-mediated event), are used as indicators of the beginning of the period of adult reproductive function. Ultimately, the manifestation of first preovulatory GnRH/LH surge (females) harbors the first ovulation. In males, the first presence of viable sperm in ejaculate is a sign of adult maturity.

A considerable body of work suggests that pubertal timing is strongly influenced by the environment as a whole, and to environmental endocrine disruptors specifically. In females, estrogenic endocrine disruptors such as bisphenol A, methoxychlor (a pesticide), PCBs, and phytoestrogens are often associated with accelerated (early) timing of puberty. In males, pubertal timing is often delayed due to actions of anti-androgenic endocrine disruptors including phthalates and vinclozolin (a fungicide). In most of these studies, the question of whether the aberrant pubertal timing was due to EDC effects on the GnRH system, or its afferent inputs, was not studied. However, considering the key role of GnRH in the timing of puberty, this is likely to be the case.

Organochlorine pesticides such as methoxychlor interfere with the process of puberty in a sex-dependent manner. When pregnant rat dams were treated with methoxychlor, their offspring exhibited advanced female puberty and delayed male puberty (Masutomi et al., 2003). Our laboratory made a similar finding for gestational exposure to estrogenic PCB mixtures (Dickerson et al., 2011b).

It is difficult to draw commonalities from effects of developmental EDC exposures, as the nature and the timing of exposures, doses, sex of the animal, and many other experimental variables will affect the outcomes [see (Diamanti-Kandarakis and Gore, 2011) for much more information on EDCs and puberty]. However, in broad strokes, EDC exposures tend to be associated with the advancement of puberty in females and a delay or no effect in males. The explanations for these sex differences are undoubtedly complex, but they include the fact that many EDCs are estrogenic—which would accelerate puberty in females, but have no effect or cause a delay in males. In addition, other EDCs are anti-androgenic—causing a delay in males but not having much effect in females. These data in experimental animals are very interesting when put into the context of the human literature. A secular trend for early puberty in girls—but not boys—has been supported by a series of carefully conducted studies in human populations (Biro et al., 2010). While many factors may contribute to this difference including improved nutrition and health care, the fact that girls, but not boys, undergo early puberty suggest that environmental exposures to xenoestrogens and/or anti-androgens may play a part in this trend.

5.2.5.2 Kisspeptin Neurons Are Potential Targets for Developmental EDCs.   Within the last decade, the neuropeptide kisspeptin was implicated as a critical regulator of GnRH neurons, playing important roles in postnatal development and the onset of puberty (Bellingham et al., 2009; Chan et al., 2009). More recently, kisspeptin has been postulated as a sensitive target of developmental endocrine disruption (Tena-Sempere, 2010). In all mammals studied to date, actions of kisspeptin on its receptor (called the Kiss1 receptor or GPR54) are crucial for the timing of puberty. From the EDC perspective, recent papers show that estrogenic EDC exposures during the perinatal period not only alter the timing of puberty but also appear to involve mediation of kisspeptin signaling in the hypothalamus. For example, the phytoestrogen genistein advances the timing of puberty in female rats, an effect accompanied by decreases in kisspeptin neural fiber density in hypothalamus together with a lack of activation of GnRH neurons during the expected GnRH/LH surge (Patisaul et al., 2009). Similarly, work published by our own laboratory showed that prenatal PCB exposure to rats, resulted in a greatly diminished hypothalamic kisspeptin network and decreased GnRH activation during the preovulatory GnRH/LH surge (Dickerson et al., 2011b). Finally, neonatal bisphenol A exposure decreased hypothalamic gene expression of kisspeptin in the peripubertal male and female rats(Tena-Sempere, 2010). These results on kisspeptin are important because the kisspeptinergic input to the GnRH neurosecretory system is thought to be critically important in mediating feedback from endogenous steroid hormones—and may be a biological target of hormonally acting xenobiotics such as environmental EDCs.

5.3   SUMMARY AND CONCLUSIONS

The nervous and endocrine systems work in concert to facilitate communication with and responses to an organism's environment. These processes allow an individual to maintain homeostasis of bodily functions and to enable reproductive capacity during times when the environment is favorable for reproductive success. The primary driving force for reproductive function is the GnRH neurosecretory system, the control of which is sexually dimorphic. By virtue of the sensitivity of GnRH neurons to endogenous hormone signals, this neurosecretory system is susceptible to the action of hormonally active EDCs, as shown by a number of *in vitro* and *in vivo* studies. Disrupted GnRH signaling may manifest as aberrations in the timing of puberty, female reproductive cycles, and reproductive senescence, among others. Whether these observed effects are due to EDC actions directly on the GnRH system, or indirectly via its afferent inputs, is not fully understood. Results from a series of human puberty studies parallel those of animal studies, with a trend for early puberty in girls—but not boys, a phenomenon that may be related to exposure to estrogenic EDCs.

. . . .

CHAPTER 6

Epigenetic Effects of EDCs

6.1   MOLECULAR EPIGENETIC MECHANISMS: AN INTRODUCTION

Because early life is a vulnerable period for perturbations by EDCs, this raises the question of the molecular mechanisms by which exposures to EDCs during these life stages may cause reprogramming of target systems. This concept requires a basic understanding of molecular epigenetics (Faulk and Dolinoy, 2011; Walker and Gore, 2011). Epigenetic programming refers to modifications to the genome (DNA), independent of actual mutations (changes in the DNA sequence). Rather, there are structural/functional modifications to other physical aspects of DNA and its interaction with cellular proteins that change the probability of whether or not a gene will be expressed. Epigenetic modifications are a critical part of the gene × environment interaction because they involve physical (e.g., conformational) changes to DNA that increase/decrease the probability of transcription, and they are also involved in RNA stability and post-transcriptional regulatory processes. These mechanisms underlie fundamental differences between cell types. For example, a neuron may express a specific set of genes that are transcribed to proteins involved in the neuron's structure and function related to neurotransmission. By contrast, a cell in your skin expresses those genes related to structure and function of this organ. However, both cells contain the same DNA sequence, underscoring the point that a subset of genes in each cell is expressed, while most other genes are repressed. Even in the nervous system, neighboring cells may have very different complements of genes that might be expressed—consider a neuron sitting next-door to a glial cell. It is the epigenetic changes described below that are responsible for the individuality of gene expression within cells.

The molecular epigenetic mechanism that has been best studied for environmental EDC exposures is DNA methylation (Figure 13). This a modification to the DNA molecule by which a methyl group is covalently added to the cytosine of a CpG dinucleotide (a cytosine located 5′ to a guanine connected by a phosphodiester bond). There is a family of enzymes called DNA methyltransferases (DNMTs) that add methyl groups at the cytosine bases in a CpG site. To date, a unique DNA demethylase has not been clearly identified, but searches are underway to try to identify these molecules.

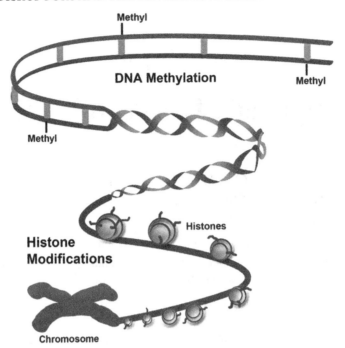

FIGURE 13: DNA methylation and histone modifications act together to regulate gene transcription. The DNA double helix is shown in blue. DNA methylation involves methyl groups added to a cytosine that is immediately 5′ to a guanine. Histone modifications involve functional groups that are added to the tails of histones (histones shown in pink, with blue tails) to change the chromatin state. Depending on the histone modification, DNA is more or less tightly wound around the histone. Modified from Qiu (2006).

    In promoters or other 5′ regulatory regions of genes, there are clusters of CpG dinucleotides that are called CpG islands. In these regions, higher levels of DNA methylation are typically associated with repression of gene expression (i.e., a "repressive mark"), whereas low levels (hypomethylation) are associated with activation of gene expression (Faulk and Dolinoy, 2011). In other parts of the DNA, e.g., introns or exonic coding regions, the relationship between DNA methylation and gene expression is often positive rather than negative, meaning that these intragenic CpG sites are not repressive (Shenker and Flanagan, 2012). DNA methylation underlies processes such as X-inactivation, imprinting of maternal or paternal genes, and tissue-specific gene expression.

    A second and well-studied molecular modification is that of histone modifications (Figure 13). There are a number of histone proteins that are involved in packaging and condensing the long strands of DNA to pack them into the nucleus. Histones are also involved in allowing this tight packaging to relax in order to reveal those regions of DNA that need to be available for expression. Histones are modified by several molecular mechanisms including acetylation, phosphorylation, ubiquitination, and methylation that control these processes. A number of enzymes have been identified that are involved in these processes.

An emerging area in epigenetic regulation is the realization that microRNAs are also important for determining stability/degradation of specific RNAs. Specific microRNAs are complementary to nucleotide sequences, usually in the 3' region of genes. Although their mechanisms are still somewhat controversial, microRNAs appear to interfere with protein translation through mRNA degradation-dependent and/or degradation-dependent events. Regardless of the mechanism, they decrease protein output from an mRNA sequence. The specificity of microRNA sequences enables them to interact with a small number of unique transcripts with complementary structure. Several miRNAs have been identified as targets for hormone signaling (Klinge, 2009), making them logical candidates for future research on EDC effects.

6.2 HORMONES AND EPIGENETIC CHANGE

There is growing evidence that the three molecular mechanisms described above are modified by steroid hormones, underscoring the key importance of epigenetics in an organism's ability to respond to the hormonal environment. A few examples of how hormones cause epigenetic change, and the relationship to sexual differentiation, follow.

6.2.1 DNA Methylation

Expression of ERα is sexually dimorphic, with levels in hypothalamus higher in adult females than males (e.g., see Figure 7). Recent research in the field of brain sexual differentiation has demonstrated that these gene expression changes are accompanied by sex differences in methylation of CpG sites in ERα gene regulatory regions (reviewed in McCarthy et al., 2009). For example, Auger's laboratory reported that the higher ERα mRNA levels in females are reflected by lower CpG methylation in the preoptic area (Kurian et al., 2010). Interestingly, this sex difference in methylation was reversed by the behavioral manipulation of increased simulated maternal grooming of the female pups. A long line of evidence has shown that maternal behavior towards pups differs for the sexes, with more licking and grooming of males than females (Weaver et al., 2004). This sex difference in exposure to maternal stimuli plays out as a whole range of phenotypic sex differences including gene and protein expression in the brain, and behavioral differences. Of relevance to the discussion on DNA methylation, it has been discovered that methylation of the ERα gene is altered by simulating maternal grooming in females (Cameron et al., 2008), work that was extended to the comparison of sex differences (Kurian et al., 2010). Thus, these lines of research on maternal behavior, sexual development, and DNA methylation have converged.

An interesting outcome of this line of work is that DNA methylation patterns are not as stable or permanent as originally thought. Two recent publications, one in cortex and one in hypothalamus, highlight this finding. In both brain regions, methylation of the ERα gene increased during postnatal life (Schwarz et al., 2010; Westberry et al., 2010), contrary to the dogma. These types of dynamic changes in methylation provide a new understanding that DNA methylation may allow more rapid environmental responses than previously thought.

6.2.2   Histone Modifications

Histone modifications are also sexually dimorphic. As an example, a comparison of markers of histone acetylation or histone methylation showed sex differences in some regions including cortex and hippocampus, but (surprisingly) not hypothalamus or amygdala (Tsai et al., 2009). In the bed nucleus of the stria terminalis of the mouse, a sexually dimorphic brain region (larger in males), a histone deacetylase inhibitor (valproic acid) given on the day of birth disrupted sexual differentiation as evidenced by smaller BNST regional volume and cell number in males or testosterone-treated masculinized females, but had no effect on normal females (Murray et al., 2009).

A recent study examined sex differences in histone acetylation in the developing preoptic area of rats and related these differences to behavioral outcomes in adulthood (Matsuda et al., 2011). That study found that binding of histone deactylase (HDAC) H2 and H4 to the ERα promoter was greater in males than in females, and there were some developmental changes. To get at the behavioral outcome, neonatal male rats were injected with a blocker of histone deacetylase. In adulthood, these males showed significant impairments in aspects of copulatory behavior.

These data suggest that developmental sex differences in histone modifications play a role in sexual differentiation of the brain. Further research is necessary in this interesting and emerging field.

6.2.3   MicroRNAs

The past decade has been an exciting one in the field of RNA research. The discovery of several new classes of RNAs has provided new insight into molecular regulatory mechanisms. MicroRNAs are a class of small non-coding RNAs that are about 20 nucleotides in length, which can interact with the 3′ untranslated regions of specific target mRNAs to affect gene expression (Klinge, 2009). Many microRNAs are encoded within introns (previously thought to be "junk" DNA). Although the mechanisms of action are not entirely understood, it is thought that by hybridizing with mRNA sequences, microRNAs can direct mRNA degradation.

Of relevance to this book, there is a growing literature showing that microRNAs regulate genes involved in hormonal regulation (e.g. through actions on ERs) and that microRNAs in turn may be regulated by steroid hormones. In hormonal cancers such as mammary cancers, microRNA expression is aberrant (Klinge, 2009). In addition, microRNAs are implicated in neurodevelopment and in adult neurobiological function (Choi et al., 2008; Miller et al., 2012). MicroRNAs are beginning to be recognized as a target for EDCs, although to our knowledge this has not yet been studied in the nervous system.

6.3 TRANSGENERATIONAL EPIGENETIC EFFECTS OF EDCs

The field of environmental epigenetics has grown by leaps and bounds in the last 5 years. By recognizing that epigenetics represents the interface between an organism's genome and its environment, scientists and public health officials are looking towards both basic research results as well as epidemiological and clinical research data in epigenetics to be able to identify problems and to develop interventions (Olden et al., 2011). Of great relevance is the discovery that some methylation marks—those that occur in the germline—may be heritable from generation to generation. This concept has become very important in the field of EDCs because it raises the concern that an exposed individual may be able to pass on an altered epigenetic state to children, grandchildren, and beyond.

Thus, work on transgenerational effects of EDCs has focused mostly on how germline methylation changes may be propagated. It is known that during embryonic development, there is a wave of demethylation and subsequently remethylation of the germline of all except the small number of maternally or paternally imprinted genes (Walker and Gore, 2011). The implications of exposure to hormones or EDCs during these phases of demethylation/remethylation include permanent changes to gene expression in that individual—and the potential for these changes to be heritable through germline transmission.

The concept of transgenerational transmission needs to consider that if exposure occurs to developing fetuses, the first unexposed generation is the F3. As shown in Figure 14, The F0 pregnant dam, when treated with an EDC during mid-gestation, exposes not only her developing F1 embryos but also the developing germ cells in the F1 animals. Those germ cells are the F2 generation, which therefore have some personal exposure to the EDC. Thus, their offspring, the F3 generation, is the first that is completely devoid of any contact with the EDC.

6.3.1 Vinclozolin

The best example of an EDC effect on heritable DNA methylation modifications comes from work published on the fungicide vinclozolin, used heavily in the wine industry. Michael Skinner's laboratory showed that when pregnant rats were exposed to vinclozolin during mid-gestation, there was no discernible effect on the pups at birth, but later in life, the males developed a host of disorders including infertility, kidney disease/cancer, testicular cancer, and other syndromes (Anway and Skinner, 2006). These effects were related to changes in DNA methylation caused by prenatal

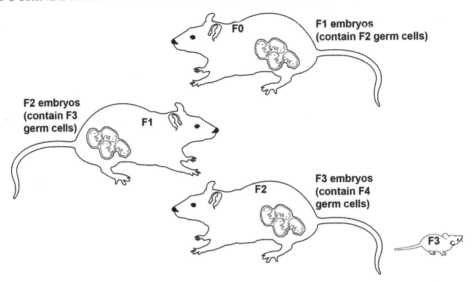

FIGURE 14: Transgenerational inheritance of epigenetic traits across 3 generations. Exposure of a pregnant dam (F0) exposes the fetal F1 offspring, as well as germ cells within the F1 that will develop into the F2 generation. The first generation completely free of any personal exposure is the F3. Modified from Walker and Gore (2011).

exposure, showing the long lapse between exposure and disease manifestation. Furthermore, this DNA methylation change was inherited in a patrilineal manner (father to son) for multiple generations, demonstrating the heritability of methylation patterns. Thus, prenatal exposure to vinclozolin causes molecular changes to the germline that are manifested for generations.

This line of research, which was initiated for studying effects on the testes, has been expanded to demonstrate that there are transgenerational epigenetic neurobiological consequences of ancestral vinclozolin exposure. A collaborative set of studies among the Skinner, Crews, and Gore labs showed that male and female rats descended from the originally exposed rats—the F3 generation (great-grandchildren) exhibited profoundly altered behaviors related to reproduction, learning and memory, and anxiety and stress (Crews et al., 2007; Skinner et al., 2008).

6.3.2 Bisphenol A

While extensively studied as an endocrine disruptor in exposed animals, a few studies have focused on its effects in multiple generations. Fertility was compromised in three generations of male rats when the pregnant or lactating dam was exposed to BPA, and expression of several hormone receptors and co-regulators was decreased in the testes across the three generations (Salian et al., 2009). Transgenerational effects of BPA on social behaviors and on gene expression of hormones/receptors involved in social behaviors (e.g., ERs, oxytocin, vasopressin) were very recently reported (Wolstenholme et al., 2012).

Although not studied in a transgenerational context, developmental BPA exposure has been shown to induce changes in DNA methylation (usually hypomethylation) in the prostate (Ho et al., 2006); DNA methylation in the forebrain of mice (Yaoi et al., 2008) and decreased DNA methylation of the agouti gene in viable yellow agouti A^{vy} mice (Dolinoy et al., 2007a). As a whole, these data show that BPA can cause molecular epigenetic changes, and together with work discussed above indicates that effects can be transmitted across generations.

6.3.3   Diethylstilbesterol (DES)

In Chapter 2, we discussed the tragedy of exposure of pregnant women—and thus their fetuses—to the estrogenic pharmaceutical, DES. Because these exposures occurred in the mid-20th century, the individuals who were exposed as fetuses are now in their 40s through 60s, and many of them had children and now grandchildren. Female children (the F1 generation) had increased reproductive abnormalities and higher propensity to develop vaginocervical carcinoma (Herbst et al., 1971). Although sample sizes of the grandchildren (F2 generation) are still small, a small but significant increase in birth defects, heart conditions, abnormalities in menstrual cycles, and a reduction in live births, have been reported [reviewed in (Walker and Gore, 2011)]. In sons of DES mothers (F1 generation), there was an increased risk of hypospadias (Klip et al., 2001). These data suggest the possibility for transgenerational effects of DES in humans, and as the descendants of the originally exposed women continue to be followed, more information will emerge.

The DES story has also been important because efforts to develop an animal model of DES have shown that the events that were observed in humans are also observed in rodents (McLachlan and Dixon, 1977). The reason this is important is because the field of endocrine disruption, while no longer considered controversial based on the weight of evidence (Grandjean et al., 2007; Diamanti-Kandarakis et al., 2009), has been challenged on occasion by those who contend that laboratory animal models are not relevant to humans. We (the authors) firmly believe that the biological processes of reproduction and other endocrine function are highly conserved—and the DES work lends credence to this belief.

As an example of the parallels between species, DES administration to pregnant rodents caused changes to the reproductive tract (uterus in females, cryoptorchidism in males). Recently, work on the F2 generation of mice showed effects in both males (lesions in the testis; reduced serum hormones) and females (increased adenocarcinoma and other reproductive tract abnormalities) (Newbold et al., 1998; Newbold et al., 2000).

Some molecular epigenetic effects of DES, particularly to DNA methylation, have been re-vealed through animal research. Perinatal exposure of mice to DES caused demethylation of the promoter of the lactoferrin gene in the uterus, paralleled by changes in gene expression (Li et al., 1997; Newbold et al., 2006). Prenatal DES exposure in mice caused changes to the uterus that were accompanied by altered expression of the HOX10A gene (involved in proper patterning of the uterus) (Bromer et al., 2009). Other effects of DES on gene expression, DNA methylation, and histone modifications have been found [reviewed in (Walker and Gore, 2011)]. Thus, while most of this work has been done in animals exposed during perinatal development (the F1 generation), re-sults provide insights into molecular mechanisms altered by DES—some of which may be heritable to future generations and underlie the effects seen across generations of humans.

6.3.4 Polychlorinated Biphenyls (PCBs)

PCB effects on molecular epigenetic endpoints on transgenerational effects have not been exten-sively studied. Our group showed that exposure of a pregnant rat to low-dose PCBs caused changes to physiology and behavior in the F1 females and had effects on hormones across the reproductive cycle of F2 rats (Steinberg et al., 2007; Steinberg et al., 2008). Another group published evidence that expression of DNA methyltransferases (which are responsible for methylation of CpG sites of target genes) was altered by PCBs, as measured in the hypothalamus and liver (Desaulniers et al., 2005; Desaulniers et al., 2009).

6.3.5 Methoxychlor

The pesticide methoxychlor is an estrogenic endocrine disruptor shown to have a range of adverse effects on reproductive systems (Zama and Uzumcu, 2010). The Uzumcu lab (Rutgers University) has carefully characterized the ovarian effects of methoxychlor following developmental exposure and has shown perturbations of ovarian development, expression of ERs in specific ovarian cell types, impaired follicular development, and other detrimental outcomes. Of relevance to this chap-ter, that lab showed that methoxychlor caused hypermethylation of the ERβ promoter, as well as 10 additional ovarian genes (Zama and Uzumcu, 2009). Moreover, expression of DNA methyltrans-ferases 3b was up-regulated, possibly explaining the hypermethylation of ERβ.

In collaboration with the Uzumcu lab, our group evaluated effects of perinatal methoxychlor exposure on reproductive aging, expression of hypothalamic genes, and underlying DNA methyla-tion changes associated with these processes (Gore et al., 2011). Female rats underwent premature reproductive aging, had abnormal hormone levels (especially serum estradiol) and had aberrant expression of a suite of genes—especially the genes for ERα and kisspeptin. Analysis of methyla-tion of CpG sites in regulatory regions of the ERα gene showed that DNA methylation was significantly up-regulated in the endocrine disrupted rats. That study, therefore, links a physiological outcome of reproductive failure and concomitant hormonal abnormalities to hypothalamic changes and DNA hypermethylation of ERα.

6.4   THE IMPORTANCE OF CONTEXT IN ENVIRONMENTAL EPIGENETICS

The environmental context is critically important in determining whether and which epigenetic molecular changes are induced by an exposure and underlies transgenerational effects (if any) of a trait. We and others (Crews, 2008) have previously defined context-dependent epigenetic mechanisms as "those molecular changes that require the exposure of the organism to a behavioral, hormonal or social context, or the presence of a causative agent (such as an EDC), for the trait to be perpetuated the exposure must occur in each generation" (Walker and Gore, 2011). An example of epigenetic programming caused by social or behavioral context is the excellent line of work in rodents showing that variations in maternal behavior or maternal stress cause a series of epigenetic changes (DNA methylation, histone modifications) to the offspring that later are manifested as behavioral and hormonal differences in those offspring (Weaver et al., 2004). In order for these traits to be further propagated, they require further exposure to the causal behavior (e.g., subsequent offspring can lose the trait if cross-fostered to mothers that do not exhibit these variations in behavior).

By contrast, work described above for vinclozolin illustrates germline-dependent epigenetic mechanisms, as the developing male germline was directly changed in its DNA methylation pattern by the EDC exposure. Thus, further exposure to the causal agent is unnecessary for further propagation of the trait. Both context- and germline-dependent epigenetic mechanisms are similar in the underlying molecular processes (e.g., methylation of DNA) but they differ because the former (context) involves somatic cells such as those in the brain, whereas the latter (germline) must involve changes to germ cells that can be heritable.

6.5   SUMMARY AND CONCLUSIONS

Epigenetic regulation of gene expression during early life plays a major role in developmental processes such as brain sexual differentiation. Some of the most widely known and best-studied epigenetic modifications include DNA methylation, histone modifications, and microRNAs. These molecular processes are vulnerable to disruption by EDCs, which may result in alterations of gene expression patterns without changes in the actual DNA sequence, ultimately manifesting as reprogramming of target systems. Not every epigenetic effect exerted by EDC exposure is limited to the exposed generation. Indeed, in early life stages, organisms are more susceptible to heritable structure changes that can be transmitted through the germline; thus such epigenetic effects persist across several generations and are termed transgenerational. EDCs known to cause transgenerational epigenetic effects include vinclozolin, BPA, DES, PCBs, and methoxychlor. The field of environmental epigenetics, although still in its early stages, has made rapid advances in the past 5 years, which have important implications ranging from ecological and evolutionary issues to human public health.

* * * *

CHAPTER 7

EDCs, the Brain, and the Future

By affecting neurobiological and endocrine systems, and impairing reproductive functions and behaviors, EDCs can quite literally affect the survival of species. There is considerable cause for concern for the future of our planet (Crews and Gore, 2011). Realistically, we must accept that the earth is contaminated and that some of these changes are irreversible. Rather than giving up hope, though, we must respond to the new challenges by moving forward with changes in human behavior to avoid further contamination, to clean up where we can, and to continue basic research into understanding the mechanisms affected by EDCs. By understanding the molecular mechanisms, we may be able to develop some pharmaceutical, nutriceutical, or other interventions in exposed individuals or populations.

7.1   CAN EDC EFFECTS BE MITIGATED?

The fact that many organic chemicals (e.g., organohalogens) were specifically designed to be lipophilic and persistent for their original applications as industrial lubricants has made it especially difficult to rid soil and water of their contamination. Most are not biodegradable, and indeed, they bioaccumulate and biomagnify up the food chain. Thus, cleaning up contaminated environments is difficult and enormously expensive. Nevertheless, there are indications that some areas that were highly contaminated are cleaner—for example, the US Environmental Protection Agency (EPA) has a "Superfund" project designed to clean up identified hazardous waste sites in the country [http://www.epa.gov/superfund/index.htm]. Despite these laudable efforts, some of the biology discussed in Chapter 6 makes it clear that cleanup is not good enough. When exposures cause epigenetic molecular changes such as DNA methylation that affect the germline and are heritable, this means the trait will be propagated even in the absence of continued exposure to the original causal insult.

Knowing that our epigenomes have been altered means that we can look toward methods for reversing or changing these molecular actions of EDC effects on DNA methylation, histone modifications, and others. There are some promising directions. EDCs can cause changes to DNA methylation, so agents that affect methylation status are potential candidates. It is known that folic acid (folate) is a methyl donor; in fact, folate supplementation is already used for pregnant women to prevent birth defects related to neural tube closure (Chang et al., 2011). This concept has not been applied (to our knowledge) to EDC exposures in humans because most of us are exposed to a variety of EDCs throughout our lives. Nevertheless, prenatal folate may have some protective benefits for these latter effects, as well as its better-known effects on prevention of spina bifida. In fact, some results in animals provide promising support for this idea. Prenatal BPA exposure in mice caused hypomethylation of some CpG sites in target genes, an effect that was mitigated by supplementation of the maternal diet by folic acid (Dolinoy et al., 2007a). For histone modifications, the histone deacetylase blocker trichostatin A (TSA) reversed epigenetic effects of maternal behavior toward rat pups on their subsequent behaviors in adulthood and expression of genes in the hippocampus (Weaver et al., 2006).

These are early first steps in developing interventions in humans. However, it is not reasonable to treat pregnant women or children with a histone deacetylase blocker such as TSA. In this case, as well as that of folate, their actions on molecular epigenetic targets are global but not necessarily specific to a single key gene, or groups of genes. While there are known benefits of increasing methylation for genes in spina bifida, there is a question of whether this is beneficial to all genes—some of which normally would have low methylation levels and for which hypermethylation may be detrimental. The same point applies to histone acetylation, blockade of which is unlikely to be globally beneficial. What would be truly useful in human therapeutics would be first, to identify the specific targets of EDCs, and second, to be able to design treatments that specifically act upon those gene targets. These and additional ideas for the future of environmental epigenomics research (Dolinoy et al., 2007b) are summarized (Box 3). These lofty goals are probably many years in the future, and real pay-off requires considerable scientific research over the next decades.

Box 3. Needs for future research on EDCs and environmental epigenomics

- Develop a rational, tiered testing system for identifying EDCs across a range of tests beginning with molecular modeling, high-throughput in vitro assays, and ultimately, physiological systems (Schug et al., 2012)
- Identify environmental factors that affect epigenetic molecular changes (DNA methylation, histone modification, etc.)
- Identify new molecular mechanisms of action of environmental EDCs that are gene-target specific (e.g., short non-coding RNAs including microRNAs)
- Define key developmental windows of vulnerability to environmental toxicants
- Perform testing of environmentally relevant doses (e.g., low doses)
- Perform testing of relevant mixtures

7.2   WHAT CAN WE DO TO AVOID EDC EXPOSURES?

The best way to avoid a complication of EDC exposure is, of course, to avoid exposure altogether. Many alternatives already exist for products that contain known EDCs. It goes without saying that it is not possible to isolate oneself from all manufactured chemicals, nor would most people choose to do so. Nevertheless, there are lifestyle choices that can be made to reduce exposures (Table 10).

Along with avoiding exposure for oneself and one's family, it is important to avoid contributing to the problems for others. The same behaviors that protect you also protect the environment. For example, decreasing one's use of plastic disposable bottles is better for your health and also decreases the mass of non-biodegradable waste. Avoiding chemical pesticides in your garden minimizes exposure of wildlife and contamination of ground water.

TABLE 10: Minimizing chemical exposures[1]
PREVENTING EXPOSURE IN THE HOME
http://www.thegreenguide.com/gg/pdf/CleaningProducts_1.pdf
Avoid smoking
Minimize upholstering, carpeting, and drapes
Toilet bowl cleaners: avoid paradichlorobenzene
Avoid chemical pesticides; keep a clean house, plug holes that allow pest entry, and use natural pest control products (borax, red chili powder, paprika, mint)
Avoid artificial fresheners or scented candles
Clean with microfiber cloths
Use low VOC paint
Reduce exposure to radon—test for radon
Avoid mothballs—use cedar or lavender

TABLE 10: (*continued*)
PREVENTING EXPOSURE IN YOUR YARD
www.beyondpesticides.org
www.pesticide.org/factsheets.html
www.pesticideinfo.org/Index.html
http://www.epa.gov/oppfead1/Publications/Cit_Guide/citguide.pdf
Do organic gardening
Avoid herbicides, pesticides
PREVENTING EXPOSURE IN YOUR FOOD AND WATER
http://www.ewg.org/foodnews/
http://www.breastcancerfund.org/reduce-your-risk/tips/eat-live-better/
Eat fresh food (reduce canned)
Know what foods have high levels of pesticides
Eat organic when possible, and wash produce
Eat fish with lower levels of mercury and PCBs
Use a water filter (minimize disposable plastic water bottles)
Microwave in glass (avoid microwaving in plastic)
Avoid BPA in plastic containers
Avoid polystyrene, styrofoam

TABLE 10: (*continued*)
PREVENTING EXPOSURE IN PERSONAL CARE PRODUCTS
http://www.ewg.org/skindeep/
www.cosmeticsdatabase.com
www.thegreenguide
Antibacterial soap, toothpaste: avoid triclosan or triclocarban
Avoid shampoos, lotions, and cosmetics with phthalates
Avoid sunscreens with oxobenzone
PREVENTING EXPOSURE IN THE WORKPLACE
Recycle
Clean with non-toxic products
Assure proper ventilation and air quality
Follow the same rules for eating and drinking as in the home
BEING A SMART CONSUMER
http://www.prhe.ucsf.edu/prhe/tmlinks.html#consumerguide
http://householdproducts.nlm.nih.gov/
Know what is in the products you buy and use—read labels
Reduce exposures in your clothes (avoid flame retardants; choose natural untreated fibers; minimize chlorine bleach)

TABLE 10: *(continued)*
HELPFUL WEBSITES WITH INFORMATION ABOUT EXPOSURES— AND AVOIDING THEM
www.ewg.org
www.edf.org
www.prhe.ucsf.edu/prhe/toxicmatter
http://www.noharm.org/us_canada/events/foodmatters/l
www.womenshealthandenvironment.org
http://www.healthystuff.org/
http://www.plannedparenthood.org/about-us/boards-initiatives/green-choices-32516.htm

[1] Courtesy of Dr. Jerry Heindel, NIEHS.

7.3 GENERAL CONCLUSIONS

The number of environmental chemicals has grown enormously over the past 50 years. This parallels an increasing trend for the prevalence of human health conditions, including impaired fertility, reproductive system cancers, metabolic disorders such as obesity and insulin resistance, and other endocrine dysfunctions. Moreover, by acting on neurotransmitters, hormone receptors, and steroidogenic enzymes, EDCs can cause neuroendocrine disruption, cognitive impairments, and behavioral disorders. Considering that autism, ADHD, and neurobehavioral deficiencies are on the rise, it is quite possible that they have links to environmental contaminants.

The developing brain is a particularly vulnerable target for EDCs. As we have discussed throughout this book, neurobiological development is strongly influenced by endogenous steroid hormone actions on neural survival or apoptosis, resulting in sex differences in numbers of neurons in specific brain regions. Hormones also have profound effects on synaptic plasticity. During fetal development and infancy, hormones also affect the phenotype of neurons—that is, which receptors a neuron expresses on its cell surface, and what genes it expresses within the cell nucleus. Thus, it is not surprising that exposure of the developing brain to EDCs has long-lasting consequences. Moreover, many of these effects may not be observable at first, but develop over time, such as during adolescence/puberty or in adulthood.

There is a complex interplay between gene and environment that is important to understand in the context of EDCs and the developing brain. During differentiation of the nervous system, there are organizational processes that determine the ultimate structure and function of each cell. This process is regulated by epigenetic mechanisms that cause structural modifications to DNA or RNA—but not overt mutations. Molecular epigenetic processes, including DNA methylation, histone modifications, and non-coding RNAs (e.g., microRNAs), are targets for environmental perturbations. Thus, recent research shows that EDCs modify the developing brain through epigenetic molecular programming. This is a relatively young field that has great promise for understanding how EDCs work, but also, in developing therapeutic interventions to some of these processes.

There is no longer any doubt that humans are exposed to, and affected by EDCs. The developing human brain is probably the most complex of all species, and therefore, the most difficult to understand. Nevertheless, the conservation of endocrine and neurobiological hormones and signaling molecules underscores the similarity across vertebrate classes. Therefore, we believe that the Precautionary Principle must be used when considering introduction of any chemical into products that come into contact with food, water, and children's clothes and toys. This principle advocates for identification of possible toxic or endocrine-disrupting properties *before*, rather than *after*, the release of such a product. That way, damage is averted and does not have to be un-done.

Although it is impossible to avoid EDC exposure entirely, recent advancements in the field of endocrine disruption and green chemistry make it possible to envision a future where EDC exposure is far more limited as a result of the cooperative action of the general public, government and chemical companies.

      . . . . .

Acknowledgments

Work described in this book from our own laboratory was generously supported by National Institutes of Health (NIEHS)1RO1 ES020662, 1RC1 ES018139 to ACG, and the National Science Foundation NSF 04-615 to SMD. We thank members of the Gore Lab for helpful conversations on these topics, and acknowledge Belinda Lehmkuhle for assistance with figures. Finally, we are grateful to Dr. Margaret M. McCarthy for inviting us to participate in this important e-book series, and to editorial staff, especially Joseph Cho, for patience and encouragement.

References

Aloisi AM, Della Seta D, Ceccarelli I and Farabollini F. 2001. Bisphenol-A differently affects estrogen receptors-alpha in estrous-cycling and lactating female rats. *Neurosci Lett* 310: pp. 49–52.

Anway MD and Skinner MK. 2006. Epigenetic transgenerational actions of endocrine disruptors. *Endocrinology* 147: pp. S43–9.

Aoki Y. 2001. Polychlorinated biphenyls, polychlorinated dibenzo-p-dioxins, and polychlorinated dibenzofurans as endocrine disrupters—what we have learned from Yusho disease. *Environ Res* 86: pp. 2–11.

Bakker J and Baum MJ. 2008. Role for estradiol in female-typical brain and behavioral sexual differentiation. *Front Neuroendocrinol* 29: pp. 1–16.

Bakker J, DeMees C, Douhard Q, Balthazart J, Gabant P, Szpirer J and Szpirer C. 2006. Alpha-fetoprotein protects the developing female mouse brain from masculinization and defeminization by estrogens. *Nat Neurosci* 9: pp. 220–6.

Barker DJ. 2003. The developmental origins of adult disease. *Eur J Epidemiol* 18: pp. 733–6.

Bateman HL and Patisaul HB. 2008. Disrupted female reproductive physiology following neonatal exposure to phytoestrogens or estrogen specific ligands is associated with decreased GnRH activation and kisspeptin fiber density in the hypothalamus. *Neurotoxicol* 29: pp. 988–97.

Bellingham M, Fowler PA, Amezaga MR, Rhind SM, Cotinot C, Mandon-Pepin B, Sharpe RM and Evans NP. 2009. Exposure to a complex cocktail of environmental endocrine-disrupting compounds disturbs the kisspeptin/GPR54 system in ovine hypothalamus and pituitary gland. *Environ Health Perspect* 117: pp. 1556–62.

Biro FM, Galvez MP, Greenspan LC, Succop PA, Vangeepuram N, Pinney SM, Teitelbaum S, Windham GC, Kushi LH and Wolff MS. 2010. Pubertal assessment method and baseline characteristics in a mixed longitudinal study of girls. *Pediatrics* 126: pp. e583–90.

Bisenius ES, Veeramachaneni DN, Sammonds GE and Tobet S. 2006. Sex differences and the development of the rabbit brain: effects of vinclozolin. *Biol Reprod* 75: pp. 469–76.

Bliss TVP and Collingridge GL. 1993. A synaptic model of memory: long-term potentiation in the hippocampus. *Nature* 361: pp. 31–9.

Bromer JG, Wu J, Zhou Y and Taylor HS. 2009. Hypermethylation of homeobox A10 by in utero diethylstilbestrol exposure: an epigenetic mechanism for altered developmental programming. *Endocrinology* 150: pp. 3376–82.

Calafat AM and Needham LL. 2007. Human exposures and body burdens of endocrine-disrupting chemicals. In: Gore AC (ed), Endocrine-Disrupting Chemicals: From Basic Research to Clinical Practice. Humana Press, Totowa, NJ, pp. 253–68.

Cameron NM, Shahrokh D, Del Corpo A, Dhir SK, Szyf M, Champagne FA and Meaney MJ. 2008. Epigenetic programming of phenotypic variations in reproductive strategies in the rat through maternal care. *J Neuroendocrinol* 20: pp. 795–801.

Chan YM, Broder-Fingert S and Seminara SB. 2009. Reproductive functions of kisspeptin and Gpr54 across the life cycle of mice and men. *Peptides* 30: pp. 42–8.

Chang H, Zhang T, Zhang Z, Bao R, Fu C, Wang Z, Bao Y, Li Y, Wu L, Zheng X and Wu J. 2011. Tissue-specific distribution of aberrant DNA methylation associated with maternal low-folate status in human neural tube defects. *J Nutr Biochem* 22: pp. 1172–7.

Choi PS, Zakhary L, Choi WY, Caron S, Alvarez-Saavedra E, Miska EA, McManus M, Harfe B, Giraldez AJ, Horvitz HR, Schier AF and Dulac C. 2008. Members of the miRNA-200 family regulate olfactory neurogenesis. *Neuron* 57: pp. 41–55.

Colciago A, Casati L, Mornati O, Vergoni AV, Santagostino A, Celotti F and Negri-Cesi P. 2009. Chronic treatment with polychlorinated biphenyls (PCB) during pregnancy and lactation in the rat. Part 2: Effects on reproductive parameters, on sex behavior, on memory retention and on hypothalamic expression of aromatase and 5alpha-reductases in the offspring. *Toxicol Appl Pharmacol* 239: pp. 46–54.

Connors SL, Levitt P, Matthews SG, Slotkin TA, Johnston MV, Kinney HC, Johnson WG, Dailey RM and Zimmerman AW. 2008. Fetal mechanisms in neurodevelopmental disorders. *Pediatr Neurol* 38: pp. 163–76.

Crews D. 2008. Epigenetics and its implications for behavioral neuroendocrinology. *Front Neuroendocrinol* 29: pp. 344–57.

Crews D and Gore AC. 2011. Life imprints: Living in a contaminated world. *Environ Health Perspect* 119: pp. 1208–10.

Crews D, Gore AC, Hsu TS, Dangleben NL, Spinetta M, Schallert T, Anway MD and Skinner MK. 2007. Transgenerational epigenetic imprints on mate preference. *Proc Natl Acad Sci USA* 104: pp. 5942–6.

Desaulniers D, Cooke GM, Leingartner K, Soumano K, Cole J, Yang J, Wade M and Yagminas A. 2005. Effects of postnatal exposure to a mixture of polychlorinated biphenyls, p,p′-dichlorodiphenyltrichloroethane, and p-p′-dichlorodiphenyldichloroethene in prepubertal and adult female Sprague–Dawley rats. *Int J Toxicol* 24: pp. 111–27.

Desaulniers D, Xiao GH, Lian H, Feng YL, Zhu J, Nakai J and Bowers WJ. 2009. Effects of mixtures of polychlorinated biphenyls, methylmercury, and organochlorine pesticides on hepatic DNA methylation in prepubertal female Sprague–Dawley rats. *Int J Toxicol* 28: pp. 294–307.

Diamanti-Kandarakis E, Bourguignon JP, Giudice LC, Hauser R, Prins GS, Soto AM, Zoeller RT and Gore AC. 2009. Endocrine-disrupting chemicals: an Endocrine Society scientific statement. *Endocr Rev* 30: pp. 293–342.

Diamanti-Kandarakis E and Gore AC. 2011. Endocrine Disruptors and Puberty. Springer/Humana Press, Totowa, NJ.

Dickerson SM, Cunningham SL and Gore AC. 2011a. Prenatal PCBs disrupt early neuroendocrine development of the rat hypothalamus. *Toxicol Appl Pharmacol* 252: pp. 36–46.

Dickerson SM, Cunningham SL, Patisaul HB, Woller MJ and Gore AC. 2011b. Endocrine disruption of brain sexual differentiation by developmental PCB exposure. *Endocrinology* 152: pp. 581–94.

Dickerson SM, Cunningham SL and Gore AC. 2012. Reproductive neuroendocrine targets of developmental exposure to endocrine disruptors. In: Diamanti-Kandarakis E and Gore AC (eds), Endocrine Disruptors and Puberty. Humana/Springer Press, Totowa, NJ.

Dingemans MM, van den Berg M and Westerink RH. 2011. Neurotoxicity of brominated flame retardants: (in)direct effects of parent and hydroxylated polybrominated diphenyl ethers on the (developing) nervous system. *Environ Health Perspect* 119: pp. 900–7.

Dolinoy DC, Huang D and Jirtle RL. 2007a. Maternal nutrient supplementation counteracts bisphenol A-induced DNA hypomethylation in early development. *Proc Natl Acad Sci* 104: pp. 13056–61.

Dolinoy DC, Weidman JR and Jirtle RL. 2007b. Epigenetic gene regulation: linking early developmental environment to adult disease. *Reprod Toxicol* 23: pp. 297–307.

Dyer CA. 2007. Heavy metals as endocrine-disrupting chemicals. In: Gore AC (ed), Endocrine-Disrupting Chemicals: From Basic Research to Clinical Practice. Humana Press, Totowa, NJ.

Erskine MS, Lehmann ML, Cameron NM and Polston EK. 2004. Co-regulation of female sexual behavior and pregnancy induction: an exploratory synthesis. *Behav Brain Res* 153: pp. 295–315.

Faulk C and Dolinoy DC. 2011. Timing is everything: the when and how of environmentally induced changes in the epigenome of animals. *Epigenetics* 6: pp. 791–7.

Fernandez M, Bianchi M, Lux-Lantos V and Libertun C. 2009. Neonatal exposure to bisphenol a alters reproductive parameters and gonadotropin releasing hormone signaling in female rats. *Environ Health Perspect* 117: pp. 757–62.

Forger NG. 2006. Cell death and sexual differentiation of the nervous system. *Neuroscience* 138: pp. 929–38.

Gore AC. 2002. GnRH: The Master Molecule of Reproduction. Kluwer Academic Publishers, Norwell, MA.

Gore AC. 2007. Endocrine-Disrupting Chemicals: From Basic Research to Clinical Practice. Humana Press, Totowa.

Gore AC. 2008. Developmental programming and endocrine disruptor effects on reproductive neuroendocrine systems. *Front Neuroendocrinol* 29: pp. 358–74.

Gore AC, Walker DM, Zama AM, Armenti AE and Uzumcu M. 2011. Early life exposure to endocrine-disrupting chemicals causes lifelong molecular reprogramming of the hypothalamus and premature reproductive aging. *Mol Endocrinol* 25: pp. 2157–68.

Grandjean P, Bellinger D, Bergman A, Cordler S, Davey-Smith G, Eskenazi B, Gee D, Gray K, Hanson M, van den Hazel P, Heindel JJ, Heinzow B, Hertz-Picciotto I, Hu H, Huang TT-K, Jensen TK, Landrigan PJ, McMillen IC, Murata K, Ritz B, Schoeters G, Skakkebaek N, Skerfving S and Weihe P. 2007. The Faroes Statement: Human health effects of developmental exposure to chemicals in our environment. *Basic Clin Pharmacol Toxicol* 102: pp. 73–5.

Grandjean P and Landrigan P. 2006. Developmental neurotoxicity of industrial chemicals. *The Lancet* 368: pp. 2167–78.

Guillette LJ, Jr., Gross TS, Masson GR, Matter JM, Percival HF and Woodward AR. 1994. Developmental abnormalities of the gonad and abnormal sex hormone concentrations in juvenile alligators from contaminated and control lakes in Florida. *Environ Health Perspect* 102: pp. 680–8.

Hajszan T and Leranth C. 2010. Bisphenol A interferes with synaptic remodeling. *Front Neuroendocrinol* 31: pp. 519–30.

Hao J, Janssen WGM, Tang Y, Roberts JA, McKay H, Lasley B, Allen PB, Greengard P, Rapp PR, Kordower JH, Hof PR and Morrison JH. 2003. Estrogen increases the number of spinophilin-immunoreactive spines in the hippocampus of young and aged female rhesus monkeys. *J Comp Neurol* 465: pp. 540–50.

Henry LA and Witt DM. 2006. Effects of neonatal resveratrol exposure on adult male and female reproductive physiology and behavior. *Devel Neurosci* 28: pp. 186–95.

Herbst AL, Ulfelder H and Poskanzer DC. 1971. Adenocarcinoma of the vagina. Association of maternal stilbestrol therapy with tumor appearance in young women. *N Engl J Med* 284: pp. 878–81.

Hites RA, Foran JA, Carpenter DO, Hamilton MC, Knuth BA and Schwager SJ. 2004. Global assessment of organic contaminants in farmed salmon. *Science* 303: pp. 226–9.

Ho SM, Tang WY, Belmonte de Frausto J and Prins GS. 2006. Developmental exposure to estradiol and bisphenol A increases susceptibility to prostate carcinogenesis and epigenetically regulates phosphodiesterase type 4 variant 4. *Cancer Res* 66: pp. 5624–32.

Ikeda M, Mitsui T, Setani K, Tamura M, Kakeyama M, Sone H, Tohyama C and Tomita T. 2005. In utero and lactational exposure to 2,3,7,8-tetrachlorodibenzo-p-dioxin in rats disrupts brain sexual differentiation. *Toxicol Appl Pharmacol* 205: pp. 98–105.

Ishido M, Morita M, Oka S and Masuo Y. 2005. Alteration of gene expression of G protein-coupled receptors in endocrine disruptors-caused hyperactive rats. *Regul Pept* 126: pp. 145–53.

Jacobson JL and Jacobson SW. 1996. Intellectual impairment in children exposed to polychlorinated biphenyls in utero. *N Engl J Med* 335: pp. 783–9.

Jobling S and Sumpter JP. 1993. Detergent components in sewage effluent are weakly oestrogenic to fish: An in vitro study using rainbow trout (Oncorhynchus mykiss) hepatocytes. *Aquat Toxicol* 27: pp. 361–72.

Jones DC and Miller GW. 2008. The effects of environmental neurotoxicants on the dopaminergic system: A possible role in drug addiction. *Biochem Pharmacol* 76: pp. 569–81.

Kauffman AS, Gottsch ML, Roa J, Byquist AC, Crown A, Clifton DK, Hoffman GE, Steiner RA and Tena-Sempere M. 2007. Sexual differentiation of Kiss1 gene expression in the brain of the rat. *Endocrinology* 148: pp. 1774–83.

Kermath BA and Gore AC. 2012. Neuroendocrine control of the transition to reproductive senescence: Lessons learned from the female rodent model. *Neuroendocrinology*.

Klinge CM. 2009. Estrogen regulation of microRNA expression. *Curr Genomics* 10: pp. 169–83.

Klip H, Burger CW, de Kraker J and van Leeuwen FE. 2001. Risk of cancer in the offspring of women who underwent ovarian stimulation for IVF. *Hum Reprod* 16: pp. 2451–8.

Kuiper GG, Lemmen JG, Carlsson B, Corton JC, Safe SH, van der Saag PT, van der Burg B and Gustafsson JA. 1998. Interaction of estrogenic chemicals and phytoestrogens with estrogen receptor beta. *Endocrinology* 139: pp. 4252–63.

Kurian JR, Olesen KM and Auger AP. 2010. Sex differences in epigenetic regulation of the estrogen receptor-alpha promoter within the developing preoptic area. *Endocrinology* 151: pp. 2297–305.

Lein PJ, Yang D, Bachstetter AD, Tilson HA, Harry GJ, Mervis RF and Kodavanti PR. 2007. Ontogenetic alterations in molecular and structural correlates of dendritic growth after developmental exposure to polychlorinated biphenyls. *Environ Health Perspec* 115: pp. 556–63.

Leranth C, Hajszan T, Szigeti-Buck K, Bober J and MacLusky NJ. 2008. Bisphenol A prevents the synaptogenic response to estradiol in hippocampus and prefrontal cortex of ovariectomized nonhuman primates. *Proc Natl Acad Sci* 105: pp. 14187–91.

Lewis RW, Brooks N, Milburn GM, Soames A, Stone S, Hall M and Ashby J. 2003. The effects of the phytoestrogen genistein on the postnatal development of the rat. *Toxicol Sci* 71: pp. 74–83.

Li S, Washburn KA, Moore R, Uno T, Teng C, Newbold RR, McLachlan JA and Negishi M. 1997.

Developmental exposure to diethylstilbestrol elicits demethylation of estrogen-responsive lactoferrin gene in mouse uterus. *Cancer Res* 57: pp. 4356–9.

Lichtensteiger W, Faass O, Ma R and Schlumpf M. 2003. Effect of polybrominated diphenylether and PCB on the development of the brain–gonadal axis and gene expression in rats. *Organohalog Compd* 61: pp. 84–7.

Luoma J. 2005. Challenged Conceptions: Environmental Chemicals and Fertility. Proceedings of "Understanding Environmental Contaminants and Human Ferility: Science and Strategy."

Markman S, Leitner S, Catchpole C, Barnsley S, Muller CT, Pascoe D and Buchanan KL. 2008. Pollutants increase song complexity and the volume of the brain area HVC in a songbird. *PLoS ONE* 3: pp. 1–6.

Masuo Y, Morita M, Oka S and Ishido M. 2004. Motor hyperactivity caused by a deficit in dopaminergic neurons and the effects of endocrine disruptors: a study inspired by the physiological roles of PACAP in the brain. *Regul Pept* 123: pp. 225–34.

Masutomi N, Shibutani M, Takagi H, Uneyama C, Takahashi N and Hirose M. 2003. Impact of dietary exposure to methoxychlor, genistein, or diisononyl phthalate during the perinatal period on the development of the rat endocrine/reproductive systems in later life. *Toxicol* 192: pp. 149–70.

Matsuda KI, Mori H, Nugent BM, Pfaff DW, McCarthy MM and Kawata M. 2011. Histone deacetylation during brain development is essential for permanent masculinization of sexual behavior. *Endocrinology* 152: pp. 2760–7.

McCarthy MM. 2011. Sex and the Developing Brain. Morgan & Claypool Life Sciences.

McCarthy MM, Auger AP, Bale TL, De Vries GJ, Dunn GA, Forger NG, Murray EK, Nugent BM, Schwarz JM and Wilson ME. 2009. The epigenetics of sex differences in the brain. *J Neurosci* 29: pp. 12815–23.

McEwen BS, Coirini H, Westlind-Danielsson A, Frankfurt M, Gould E, Schumacher M and Woolley C. 1991. Steroid hormones as mediators of neural plasticity. *Steroid Biochem Molec Biol* 39: pp. 223–32.

McLachlan JA and Dixon RL. 1977. Toxicologic comparison of experimental and clinical exposure to diethylstilbestrol during gestation. *Adv Sex Steroid Horm Res* 3: pp. 309–36.

Mellon PL, Windle JJ, Goldsmith PC, Padula CA, Roberts JL and Weiner RI. 1990. Immortalization of hypothalamic GnRH neurons by genetically targeted tumorigenesis. *Neuron* 5: pp. 1–10.

Miller BH, Zeier Z, Xi L, Lanz TA, Deng S, Strathmann J, Willoughby D, Kenny PJ, Elsworth JD, Lawrence MS, Roth RH, Edbauer D, Kleiman RJ and Wahlestedt C. 2012. MicroRNA-132 dysregulation in schizophrenia has implications for both neurodevelopment and adult brain function. *Proc Natl Acad Sci U S A* 109: pp. 3125–30.

Moniz AC, Cruz-Casallas PE, Salzgeber SA, Varoli FMF, Spinosa HS and Bernardi MM. 2005. Behavioral and endocrine changes induced by perinatal fenvalerate exposure in female rats. *Neurotoxicol Teratol* 27: pp. 609–14.

Monje L, Varayoud J, Luque EH and Ramos JG. 2007. Neonatal exposure to bisphenol A modifies the abundance of estrogen receptor a transcripts with alternative 50-untranslated regions in the female rat preoptic area. *J Endocrinol* 194: pp. 201–12.

Morrison JH, Brinton RD, Schmidt PJ and Gore AC. 2006. Estrogen, menopause, and the aging brain: how basic neuroscience can inform hormone therapy in women. *J Neurosci* 26: pp. 10332–48.

Murray EK, Hien A, de Vries GJ and Forger NG. 2009. Epigenetic control of sexual differentiation of the bed nucleus of the stria terminalis. *Endocrinology* 150: pp. 4241–7.

Newbold RR, Hanson RB, Jefferson WN, Bullock BC, Haseman J and McLachlan JA. 1998. Increased tumors but uncompromised fertility in the female descendants of mice exposed developmentally to diethylstilbestrol. *Carcinogenesis* 19: pp. 1655–63.

Newbold RR, Hanson RB, Jefferson WN, Bullock BC, Haseman J and McLachlan JA. 2000. Proliferative lesions and reproductive tract tumors in male descendants of mice exposed developmentally to diethylstilbestrol. *Carcinogenesis* 21: pp. 1355–63.

Newbold RR, Padilla-Banks E and Jefferson WN. 2006. Adverse effects of the model environmental estrogen diethylstilbestrol (DES) are transmitted to subsequent generations. *Endocrinology* 147: pp. S11–7.

Olden K, Freudenberg N, Dowd J and Shields AE. 2011. Discovering how environmental exposures alter genes could lead to new treatments for chronic illnesses. *Health Aff (Millwood)* 30: pp. 833–41.

Panzica GC, Viglietti-Panzica C, Mura E, Quinn MJJ, Lavoie E, Palanza P and Ottinger MA. 2007. Effects of xenoestrogens on the differentiation of behaviorally-relevant neural circuits. *Front Neuroendocrinol* 28: pp. 179–200.

Patisaul HB, Fortino AE and Polston EK. 2006. Neonatal genistein or bisphenol-A exposure alters sexual differentiation of the AVPV. *Neurotoxicol Teratol* 28: pp. 111–8.

Patisaul HB, Fortino AE and Polston EK. 2007. Differential disruption of nuclear volume and neuronal phenotype in the preoptic area by neonatal exposure to genistein and bisphenol-A. *Neurotoxicol* 28: pp. 1–12.

Patisaul HB and Jefferson W. 2010. The pros and cons of phytoestrogens. *Front Neuroendocrinol* 31: pp. 400–19.

Patisaul HB, Todd KL, Mickens JA and Adewale HB. 2009. Impact of neonatal exposure to the ERalpha agonist PPT, bisphenol-A or phytoestrogens on hypothalamic kisspeptin fiber density in male and female rats. *Neurotoxicol* 30: pp. 350–7.

Pesatori AC, Consonni D, Bachetti S, Zocchetti C, Bonzini M, Baccarelli A and Bertazzi PA. 2003. Short- and long-term morbidity and mortality in the population exposed to dioxin after the "Seveso Accident." *Ind Health* 41: pp. 127–38.

Plant TM. 2012. A comparison of the neuroendocrine mechanisms underlying the initiation of the preovulatory LH surge in the human, old world monkey and rodent. *Front Neuroendocrinol* (ePub).

Qiu J. 2006. Epigenetics: unfinished symphony. *Nature* 441: pp. 143–5.

Quinn CL, Wania F, Czub G and Breivik K. 2011. Investigating intergenerational differences in human PCB exposure due to variable emissions and reproductive behaviors. *Environ Health Perspect* 119: pp. 641–6.

Rasier G, Parent A-S, Gerard A, Denooz R, Lebrethon M-C, Charlier C and Bourguignon JP. 2008. Mechanisms of interaction of endocrine-disrupting chemicals with glutamate-evoked secretion of gonadotropin-releasing hormone. *Toxicol Sci* 102: pp. 33–41.

Rhees RW, Shryne JE and Gorski RA. 1990. Onset of the hormone-sensitive perinatal period for sexual differentiation of the sexually dimorphic nucleus of the preoptic area in female rats. *J Neurobiol* 21: pp. 781–6.

Salian S, Doshi T and Vanage G. 2009. Perinatal exposure of rats to Bisphenol A affects the fertility of male offspring. *Life Sci* 85: pp. 742–52.

Schantz SL and Widholm JJ. 2001. Cognitive effects of endocrine-disrupting chemicals in animals. *Environ Health Perspect* 109: pp. 1197–206.

Schug T, Abagyan R, Blumberg B, Collins T, Crews D, DeFur P, Dickerson S, Edwards T, Gore A, Guillette L, Hayes T, Heindel J, Moores A, Patisaul H, Tal T, Thayer K, Vandenberg L, Warner J, Watson C, vom Saal F, Zoeller R, O'Brien K and Myers J. 2012. Designing endocrine disruption out of the next generation of chemicals. *Green Chemistry* (under review).

Schwarz JM, Nugent BM and McCarthy MM. 2010. Developmental and hormone-induced epigenetic changes to estrogen and progesterone receptor genes in brain are dynamic across the life span. *Endocrinology* 151: pp. 4871–81.

Seegal RF. 1996. Epidemiological and laboratory evidence of PCB-induced neurotoxicity. *Crit Rev Toxicol* 26: pp. 709–37.

Sheehan DM. 2006. No threshold dose-response curves for nongenotoxic chimcals: Findings and applications for risk assessment. *Environ Res* 100: pp. 93–9.

Sheehan DM, Willingham E, Gaylor D, Bergeron JM and Crews D. 1999. No threshold dose for estradiol-induced sex reversal of turtle embryos: how little is too much? *Environm Health Perspect* 107: pp. 155–9.

Shenker N and Flanagan JM. 2012. Intragenic DNA methylation: implications of this epigenetic mechanism for cancer research. *Br J Cancer* 106: pp. 248–53.

Sherwin BB and Henry JF. 2008. Brain aging modulates the neuroprotective effects of estrogen on selective aspects of cognition in women: a critical review. *Front Neuroendocrinol* 29: pp. 88–113.

Simerly RB. 1989. Hormonal control of the development and regulation of tyrosine hydroxylase expression within a sexually dimorphic population of dopaminergic cells in the hypothalamus. *Mol Brain Res* 6: pp. 297–310.

Simerly RB. 2002. Wired for reproduction: organization and development of sexually dimorphic circuits in the mammalian forebrain. *Ann Rev Neurosci* 25: pp. 507–36.

Simerly RB, Chang C, Muramatsu M and Swanson LW. 1990. Distribution of androgen and estrogen receptor mRNA-containing cells in the rat brain: An *in situ* hybridization study. *J Comp Neurol* 294: pp. 76–95.

Simerly RB, Zee MC, Pendleton JW, Lubahn DB and Korach KS. 1997. Estrogen receptor-dependent sexual differentiation of dopaminergic neurons in the preoptic region of the mouse. *Proc Natl Acad Sci USA* 94: pp. 14077–82.

Sisk CL and Foster DL. 2004. The neural basis of puberty and adolescence. *Nature Neurosci* 7: pp. 1040–7.

Skinner MK, Anway MD, Savenkova MI, Gore AC and Crews D. 2008. Transgenerational epigenetic programming of the brain transcriptome and anxiety behavior. *PLoS ONE* 3 (e3745): pp. 1–11.

Stahlhut RW, Welshons WV and Swan SH. 2009. Bisphenol A data in NHANES suggest longer than expected half-life, substantial nonfood exposure, or both. *Environ Health Perspect* 117: pp. 784–9.

Steinberg RM, Juenger TE and Gore AC. 2007. The effects of prenatal PCBs on adult female paced mating reproductive behaviors in rats. *Horm Behav* 51: pp. 364–72.

Steinberg RM, Walker DM, Juenger TE, Woller MJ and Gore AC. 2008 Effects of perinatal polychlorinated biphenyls on adult female rat reproduction: development, reproductive physiology, and second generational effects. *Biol Reprod* 78: pp. 1091–101.

Takagi H, Shibutani M, Lee KY, Masutomi N, Fujita H, Inoue K, Mitsumori K and Hirose M. 2005. Impact of maternal dietary exposure to endocrine-acting chemicals on progesterone receptor expression in microdissected hypothalamic medial preoptic areas of rat offspring. *Toxicol Appl Pharmacol* 208: pp. 127–36.

Tando S, Itoh K, Yaoi T, Ikeda J, Fujiwara Y and Fushiki S. 2007. Effects of pre- and neonatal exposure to bisphenol A on murine brain development. *Brain Dev* 29: pp. 352–6.

Tena-Sempere M. 2010. Kisspeptin/GPR54 system as potential target for endocrine disruption of reproductive development and function. *Int J Androl* 33: pp. 360–8.

Terasawa E and Fernandez DL. 2001. Neurobiological mechanisms of the onset of puberty in primates. *Endocr Rev* 22: pp. 111–51.

Tian YH, Baek JH, Lee SY and Jang CG. 2010. Prenatal and postnatal exposure to bisphenol A induces anxiolytic behaviors and cognitive deficits in mice. *Synapse* 64: pp. 432–9.

Tsai HW, Grant PA and Rissman EF. 2009. Sex differences in histone modifications in the neonatal mouse brain. *Epigenetics* 4: pp. 47–53.

Vandenberg LN, Colborn T, Hayes TB, Heindel JJ, Jacobs DRJ, Lee D-H, Shioda T, Soto AM, vom Saal FS, Welshons WV, Zoeller RT and Myers JP. 2012. Hormones and endocrine-disrupting chemicals: low-dose effects and nonmonotonic dose responses. *Endocr Rev* 33: ePub.

vom Saal FS, Akingbemi BT, Belcher SM, Birnbaum LS, Crain DA, Eriksen M, Farabollini F, Guillette LJ, Jr., Hauser R, Heindel JJ, Ho SM, Hunt PA, Iguchi T, Jobling S, Kanno J, Keri RA, Knudsen KE, Laufer H, LeBlanc GA, Marcus M, McLachlan JA, Myers JP, Nadal A, Newbold RR, Olea N, Prins GS, Richter CA, Rubin BS, Sonnenschein C, Soto AM, Talsness CE, Vandenbergh JG, Vandenberg LN, Walser-Kuntz DR, Watson CS, Welshons WV, Wetherill Y and Zoeller RT. 2007. Chapel Hill bisphenol A expert panel consensus statement: integration of mechanisms, effects in animals and potential to impact human health at current levels of exposure. *Reprod Toxicol* 24: pp. 131–8.

Wadas BC, Hartshorn CA, Aurand ER, Palmer JS, Roselli CE, Noel ML, Gore AC, Veeramachaneni DN and Tobet SA. 2010. Prenatal exposure to vinclozolin disrupts selective aspects of the gonadotrophin-releasing hormone neuronal system of the rabbit. *J Neuroendocrinol* 22: pp. 518–26.

Walker DM and Gore AC. 2011. Transgenerational neuroendocrine disruption of reproduction. *Nat Rev Endocrinol* 7: pp. 197–207.

Wang XQ, Fang J, Nunez AA and Clemens LG. 2002. Developmental exposure to polychlorinated biphenyls affects sexual behavior of rats. *Physiol Behav* 75: pp. 689–96.

Weaver IC, Cervoni N, Champagne FA, D'Alessio AC, Sharma S, Seckl JR, Dymov S, Szyf M and Meaney MJ. 2004. Epigenetic programming by maternal behavior. *Nat Neurosci* 7: pp. 847–54.

Weaver IC, Meaney MJ and Szyf M. 2006. Maternal care effects on the hippocampal transcriptome and anxiety-mediated behaviors in the offspring that are reversible in adulthood. *Proc Natl Acad Sci U S A* 103: pp. 3480–5.

Weiss B. 2002. Sexually dimorphic nonreproductive behaviors as indicators of endocrine disruption. *Environ Health Perspect* 110(Suppl 3):387–91.

Westberry JM, Trout AL and Wilson ME. 2010. Epigenetic regulation of estrogen receptor alpha gene expression in the mouse cortex during early postnatal development. *Endocrinology* 151: pp. 731–40.

Whitten PL, Lewis C, Russell E and Naftolin F. 1995. Phytoestrogen influences on the development of behavior and gonadotropin function. *Proc Soc Exp Biol Med* 208: pp. 82–6.

Willingham E and Crews D. 1999. Sex reversal effects of environmentally relevant xenobiotic concentrations on the red-eared slider turtle, a species with temperature-dependent sex determination. *Gen Comp Endocrinol* 113: pp. 429–35.

Wolstenholme JT, Taylor JA, Shetty SR, Edwards M, Connelly JJ and Rissman EF. 2011. Gestational exposure to low dose bisphenol A alters social behavior in juvenile mice. *PLoS ONE* 6: p. e25448.

Wolstenholme W, Edwards M, Shetty SRJ, Gatewood JD, Taylor JA, Rissman EF, Connelly JJ. 2012. Gestational exposure to bisphenol A produces trans-generational changes in behaviors and gene expression. *Endocrinology* (In Press).

Wray S. 2010. From nose to brain: Development of gonadotropin-releasing hormone-1 neurons. *J Neuroendocrinol* 22: pp. 743–53.

Yaoi T, Itoh K, Nakamura K, Ogi H, Fujiwara Y and Fushiki S. 2008. Genome-wide analysis of epigenomic alterations in fetal mouse forebrain after exposure to low doses of bisphenol A. *Biochem Biophys Res Commun* 376: pp. 563–7.

Yin W and Gore AC. 2010. The hypothalamic median eminence and its role in reproductive aging. *Ann NY Acad Sci* 1204: pp. 113–22.

Zama AM and Uzumcu M. 2009. Fetal and neonatal exposure to the endocrine disruptor methoxychlor causes epigenetic alterations in adult ovarian genes. *Endocrinology* 150: pp. 4681–91.

Zama AM and Uzumcu M. 2010. Epigenetic effects of endocrine-disrupting chemicals on female reproduction: an ovarian perspective. *Front Neuroendocrinol* 31: pp. 420–39.

Zhao R, Wang Y, Zhou Y, Ni Y, Lu L, Grossmann R and Chen J. 2004. Dietary daidzein influences laying performance of ducks (Anas platyrhynchos) and early post-hatch growth of their hatchlings by modulating gene expression. *Comp Biochem Physiol A Mol Integr Physiol* 138: pp. 459–66.

FURTHER RECOMMENDED READING

Neurotoxicity of industrial chemicals in humans: Grandjean P and Landrigan P. 2006. Developmental neurotoxicity of industrial chemicals. *The Lancet* 368: pp. 2167–78.

Cognitive effects of EDCs in animals: Schantz SL and Widholm JJ. 2001. Cognitive effects of endocrine-disrupting chemicals in animals. *Environ Health Perspect* 109: pp. 1197–206.

Overview of EDC effects on human health: Diamanti-Kandarakis E, Bourguignon JP, Giudice LC, Hauser R, Prins GS, Soto AM, Zoeller RT and Gore AC. 2009. Endocrine-disrupting chemicals: an Endocrine Society scientific statement. *Endocr Rev* 30: pp. 293–342.

Patisaul HB and Jefferson W. 2010. The pros and cons of phytoestrogens. *Front Neuroendocrinol* 31: pp. 400–19.

Hormones and brain sexual differentiation: Bakker J and Baum MJ. 2008. Role for estradiol in

female-typical brain and behavioral sexual differentiation. *Front Neuroendocrinol* 29: pp. 1–16.
McCarthy MM. 2011. Sex and the Developing Brain. Morgan & Claypool Life Sciences.

EDC effects on brain sexual differentiation: Gore AC. 2008. Developmental programming and endocrine disruptor effects on reproductive neuroendocrine systems. *Front Neuroendocrinol* 29: pp. 358–74.

Book on GnRH neurons: Gore AC. 2002. GnRH: The Master Molecule of Reproduction. Kluwer Academic Publishers, Norwell, MA.

Book on basic and clinical research into environmental EDCs: Gore AC. 2007. Endocrine-Disrupting Chemicals: From Basic Research to Clinical Practice. Humana Press, Totowa.

Book on EDC effects on the timing of puberty: Diamanti-Kandarakis E and Gore AC. 2011. Endocrine Disruptors and Puberty. Springer/Humana Press, Totowa, NJ.

Author Biographies

Dr. Andrea Gore is the Gustavus and Louise Pfeiffer Professor of Pharmacology and Toxicology at the University of Texas at Austin. Dr. Gore was educated at Princeton University (BA—Biology), University of Wisconsin-Madison (PhD—Neuroscience), and Mount Sinai School of Medicine (Postdoctoral Fellow—Molecular Neuroendocrinology). Dr. Gore's NIH-funded research focuses on how the nervous system controls reproductive hormones and how the body's hormones in turn feed back to the brain to regulate neurobiological functions. Ongoing studies are investigating the links between estrogen and the aging brain during menopause. In addition, Dr. Gore's lab has been studying how environmental contaminants may perturb the body's hormonal systems and affect neurobiological development and aging. Outside of the laboratory, Dr. Gore is involved in scientific and community organizations, particularly related to mentorship, career development, and dissemination of scientific knowledge. She has received a number of citations for her work, including the Faculty Council 2001 Award for Academic Excellence (Mount Sinai School of Medicine), the University of Texas Cooperative's 2008 Research Excellent Award for Best Research Paper, and election as Fellow to the American Association for the Advancement of Science (AAAS).

Dr. Sarah Dickerson is currently a Post Doctorate Research Associate at Advancing Green Chemistry. Dr. Dickerson was educated at Sam Houston State University (BS—Biology) and the University of Texas at Austin (PhD—Toxicology). Her research interests include the impact of endocrine disrupting chemicals on development of brain regions that control reproduction. She has received national recognition for her graduate research, including a Young Investigator Award from Women in Endocrinology, an Endocrine Scholars Award from The Endocrine Society, and a Graduate Research Fellowship from the National Science Foundation.